THE TYPE
ZERO
DIABETIC

My Journey as Patient Zero

DR. HORMONE HACKER

ISBN: 978-1-968061-69-2

Table of Contents

The Zero Effect

In a world where zero often signifies absence or failure, I'm about to flip the script. When it comes to diabetes, zero isn't just a goal—it's a triumph. Welcome to the journey of becoming a Type Zero diabetic, where every step towards zero is a step towards vibrant health and longevity.

This book is your dose of reality—the truth you might not be getting from your current healthcare provider. We're going to evolve you from a Type U diabetic—Unknown, Undiagnosed, or just plain Unaware—to a Type Zero champion.

Here's what you will learn:

- My personal journey as a prediabetic and the fight to overcome my family history
- How and why I became Dr. Hormone Hacker
- The sustainable lifestyle to prevent diabetes

My promise to you? To empower you with the tools to become a Type Zero diabetic. It's about understanding your body, making informed choices, and taking control of your health destiny.

This journey isn't about achieving perfection. It's about making progress, staying persistent, and embracing the transformative power of small, consistent changes. I want to help you challenge the status quo, rewrite your health story, and be in control against diabetes.

Are you ready to join the exclusive Zero club? To defy your family history and chart a new course for your health? Although it's free to join the Zero Club, know this: when you sign up, you're literally signing your name in blood. This isn't just a casual membership; it's a solemn commitment to your health and well-being. Maintaining your membership demands discipline and fierce internal motivation.

If I haven't scared you off and this resonates with you (or even just reading on with curiosity), congratulations—you've already taken the first bold step. Now, let's dive in and take control of your health destiny. Turn the page, and let's kickstart this revolution together!

CHAPTER 1

A Prescription for Change: How I Became Dr. Hormone Hacker

I remember many mornings watching my father start his day with a thick slice of Sara Lee's pound cake, topped with a heaping mound of orange marmalade, coffee in his left hand and the newspaper in his right. Seated next to him was my mother, enjoying her butter croissant dipped in what she affectionately called "coffee," which was more cream and sugar than coffee (blink if this is you).

For a long time, that's what I thought everyone ate for breakfast. Back then, we weren't bombarded with a million Instagram reels showcasing what everyone was eating every minute of the day. So, I continued blissfully indulging in excessive carbs and sweets, believing that my active lifestyle—tennis matches and workouts—would protect me from ever getting Type 2 diabetes. I mean, thin people didn't get diabetes, right?

I was the "skinny" girl in any friend group—thank you, Dad, for passing on that fast metabolism! With obesity and physical inactivity being the culprits behind 90–95% of diabetes cases in the U.S., I felt invincible. Little did I know that my family history would soon catch up with me.

Sometimes, you don't choose your destiny; your destiny chooses you. Growing up in a medical family—my father was a surgeon, my mother a pharmacist, and both my older brothers are physicians—I was determined to be a rebel. I was going to be a journalist! What I loved most about journalism was diving into people's stories on a deeper level, uncovering truths that often lay beneath the surface. But when it came time to make my career choice, the gravitational pull of my family's legacy was too strong, and I found myself joining the family business.

Endocrinology intrigued me because it allowed me to combine my love for storytelling with medicine. I thrived on engaging with diabetics—learning about their daily habits (diet and exercise) and the challenges they faced (side effects or costs of medications). Little did I know how much this career choice would impact my own life.

As I entered my 40s, a dark cloud began to loom over my family like an ominous chess game unfolding before me. One by one, relatives fell victim to diabetes—the first "check" was my beloved grandmother. I remember her standing for hours in the kitchen making my favorite Vietnamese dishes, her laughter filling the air. None of us were even aware she had diabetes until it led to a devastating stroke that confined her to her bed until she passed.

The next "check" was my aunt—the only person who would play Scrabble with me. She had to endure the grueling routine of kidney dialysis—a life-altering consequence of her long battle with diabetes. And then came the final blow: "checkmate"—my mother suffered multiple mini-strokes that chipped away at her vibrant personality and active lifestyle.

These weren't just patients or case studies; they were the women who shaped my life. Their struggles hit close to home, making the disease's impact painfully personal. As an endocrinologist, I felt helpless and guilty watching those I loved battle this relentless condition. I kept asking myself, *Could this have been prevented?*

After witnessing so many important women in my life succumb to the challenges of diabetes, a chilling realization struck me: I could be next! Maybe you've felt this, too—that moment when your family's health history suddenly becomes a mirror reflecting a future you never wanted to see.

Determined to break this cycle of disease, I set out on a quest to reclaim control over my health.

But here's where things got tricky. Despite years of medical training as an endocrinologist, I found myself drowning in an ocean of overwhelming information online—conflicting advice about nutrition and lifestyle changes that left me more confused than ever. If navigating this sea of data was challenging for me as an endocrinologist, how frustrating must it be for you?

During my fellowship at the University of Michigan, the endocrinology clinics where I trained were reactionary at best. None focused on nutrition or exercise as integral components of treatment. We were taught to prescribe medications but rarely encouraged to explore lifestyle changes that could prevent or even reverse chronic conditions.

And so I began charting my own course to reverse my prediabetes. I stayed clear of drastic measures or extreme diets; I wanted to make empowered and sustainable choices in my everyday routine. Two months later, I was shocked by the results: my A1c had dropped from 5.6 to 5.2—all without medication! The impact of my lifestyle changes (detailed in the upcoming chapters) was astonishing; they proved more effective than some prescriptions I had started my patients on.

If you're feeling overwhelmed by improving your health, let me assure you: You don't need to turn your life upside down. With the right knowledge and guidance, small steps can lead to remarkable changes.

My personal health journey transformed not only how I live my life, but also how I practice medicine. It ignited a passion within me to help others rewrite their health stories—to bridge the gap between medical knowledge and practical health habits.

As Dr. Hormone Hacker was born—not just as a title but as a mission—I realized that truly helping patients meant addressing root causes rather than merely treating symptoms. My personal experience became a turning point in my career. I understand now that clinging to unhealthy habits from my past almost led me down a path toward diseases that I saw devastate my loved ones. But here's the empowering truth: I changed my narrative, and so can you! If you've ever felt fear mixed with hope when looking at your family history, wishing for different endings, know you're not alone—I have been there! Your story isn't predetermined; it's a living narrative changing with each choice you make.

I want you to feel the hope and empowerment I've discovered because I hacked a way to rewrite my health story, breaking free from cycles of disease plaguing my family for generations. This freedom can be yours, too!

But as Nelson Mandela warned: "One cannot be prepared for something while secretly believing it will not happen." It's time we prepare ourselves for action!

Now that we're ready to take action and rewrite our health story, it's time to dive into the heart of the matter—understanding the different faces of diabetes, so we can outsmart it at every turn.

CHAPTER 2

50 Shades of Sweet: Unmasking the Different Types of Diabetes

"A correct diagnosis is three-fourths the remedy."
— Mahatma Gandhi

N ow that we've laid the groundwork for change within ourselves, it's time to formulate our plan of attack against diabetes. Understanding the enemy is crucial in any battle, and when it comes to diabetes, knowledge is your most powerful weapon. By understanding the different types, symptoms, and risk factors, you're already well on your way to taking control of your health.

Diabetes isn't just one condition; it's a spectrum of disorders that affect how your body uses insulin. Let's break down the three main types— type 1, type 2, and type 3 (YES, did you know this existed?)—so you can recognize the signs and symptoms and understand what you're up against.

1. Type 1 Diabetes

This is an autoimmune condition where your body mistakenly attacks the insulin-producing cells in your pancreas. This means you can't make your own insulin at all. It often develops in childhood or adolescence, but can occur at any age. Symptoms can include:

- Increased thirst
- Frequent urination
- Extreme fatigue
- Blurred vision
- Unintended weight loss

ATTENTION, because this could save a life. If you or someone you care about is showing signs of type 1 diabetes, don't wait around hoping it'll get better. This isn't a "wait and see" situation—it's a "get to the doctor now" emergency. We're talking about a quick blood test that could be the difference between simply starting your loved one on insulin versus a lengthy and complicated ICU stay. With type 1 diabetes, your body's insulin factory has shut down, which is potentially life-threatening. The sooner you know, the sooner you can take action. So don't hesitate—your health (or your loved one's) could be on the line.

2. Type 2 Diabetes

Now let's talk about type 2 diabetes, which is far more common and often develops later in life. It's increasingly being diagnosed in younger individuals due to rising obesity rates. In this case, your body still produces insulin but becomes resistant to its effects. Essentially, your pancreas has to work overtime to keep up with demand. Common symptoms include:

- Increased hunger
- Fatigue
- Blurred vision

- Slow-healing sores or frequent infections
- Areas of darkened skin (often in the armpits or neck)

Diagnosis usually involves blood tests that measure fasting blood sugar levels or an A1c test. According to guidelines from the American Diabetes Association, a fasting blood sugar level of 126 mg/dL or higher indicates diabetes, while an A1c level of 6.5% or higher confirms the diagnosis. These two tests should be monitored frequently, at least once every six months.

3. Type 3 Diabetes

This is a term that's gaining traction in medical discussions and refers to conditions associated with neurodegenerative diseases like Alzheimer's and Parkinson's disease. While it's not classified as a traditional type of diabetes like type 1 or type 2, it highlights the connection between insulin resistance and brain health. Symptoms can overlap with those of Alzheimer's:

- Memory loss
- Confusion
- Mood changes
- Difficulty concentrating

Diagnosis may involve cognitive assessments alongside blood sugar testing to determine how well your body processes insulin.

4. Gestational Diabetes

Gestational diabetes is a type of diabetes that develops during pregnancy in women who didn't already have diabetes. It usually shows up in the second or third trimester when pregnancy hormones interfere with how your body uses insulin. That insulin resistance leads to elevated blood sugar levels, which can affect both mom and baby. Unlike type 1 or type 2 diabetes, gestational diabetes typically goes away after delivery, but it's still a serious condition.

You might not notice any obvious symptoms, but possible signs can include:

- Increased thirst
- More frequent urination
- Fatigue
- Nausea
- Blurred vision
- Sugar in the urine (usually picked up during routine prenatal visits)

Here's the raw truth: Gestational diabetes isn't just a pregnancy hiccup—it's a wake-up call. Left unmanaged, it can lead to serious complications like high birth weight, early delivery, and long-term health risks for both you and your child. But even more importantly, it's a signpost pointing to your future: **up to 50% of women who've had gestational diabetes will develop type 2 diabetes within 5 to 10 years**, especially if they don't take action after delivery.

But here's the good news: level up and embrace Type Zero. You've just been handed a map to your future health. You can follow the old path… or you can forge a new one.

And after delivery? The mission continues. **Don't ghost your health.** Keep showing up for yourself. That's what being a Zero Club member is all about—small, relentless steps in the right direction. So, if you've had gestational diabetes, let it be your turning point—not your downfall.

Common Risk Factors

Understanding risk factors is essential for prevention. Here are some key contributors to each type:

- Type 1 Diabetes: Family history may play a role, but environmental triggers are often involved.
- Type 2 Diabetes: Obesity, sedentary lifestyle, poor diet, family history, age (especially over 45), certain ethnic backgrounds, having had gestational diabetes during pregnancy, and having a baby weighing more than 9 pounds all increase risk. Did you know that nearly 90% of people with type 2 diabetes are overweight or obese? That's a staggering statistic that underscores the importance of lifestyle choices.
- Type 3 Diabetes: Factors such as obesity, poor diet, lack of exercise, and genetic predisposition can contribute.
- Gestational Diabetes (GDM): Risk climbs if you're over 25, overweight before pregnancy, have a family history of diabetes, or belong to certain ethnic backgrounds (including African American, Hispanic, Native American, or South Asian). Previous pregnancies with GDM or delivering a baby weighing over 9 pounds? That bumps your chances, too. Polycystic ovary syndrome (PCOS) and carrying twins (or more) can also stack the odds.

The Importance of Early Diagnosis

As an endocrinologist who has witnessed the devastating effects of diabetes, I've seen firsthand, in my patients and my own family, how this disease can ravage the body and spirit. I've watched patients lose their sight, their limbs, and their independence by having to rely on a kidney dialysis machine. I've seen families torn apart by the relentless demands of managing this condition. And I refuse to let this be your future—or mine. That's why I'm here to share crucial knowledge about the urgency of early detection, knowledge that could be the difference between a life of vitality and one of constant struggle. I've dedicated my career to understanding this disease, and I'm determined to use that understanding to help you avoid the heartbreak I've seen too many times in my practice. This isn't just medical advice—it's a lifeline I'm throwing to you, because I genuinely care about your well-being and the quality of life you deserve.

You know that fasting glucose of 98 mg/dL your doctor said was "normal"? I'm here to tell you LOUD AND CLEAR, it's anything but. That number is teetering on the edge of prediabetes, which starts at 100 mg/dL. It's like standing on the edge of a cliff—one step in the wrong direction, and you could quickly free-fall into diabetes territory.

I will never forget my personal wake-up call that changed everything for me. When my A1c came back at 5.6%, that wouldn't have raised eyebrows for many healthcare providers. For me, that 5.6% was like seeing a car speeding towards me, with my grandmother's bedridden form, my aunt's dialysis sessions, and my mother's mini-strokes, all flashing before my eyes. I had a choice: I could ignore these early warning signs like so many do, or I could take action right then and there. I chose action, and I hope you will, too. Because when it comes to your health, waiting until you're in the danger zone is like waiting to put on your seatbelt until you're halfway through the windshield. Don't wait for the crash!

Now, let's talk about something mind-blowing that most people don't know. You've got these vital cells in your pancreas called beta cells (Note: in type 1 diabetes, the body's immune system mistakenly destroys the beta cells). These precious beta cells make insulin, which controls your sugar level in the blood. But take note: by the time you're just a toddler around age two, your body has already made most of the beta cells you'll ever have. Imagine being handed a piggy bank as a toddler and told, "This is it, kid. Make it last a lifetime." That's essentially what's happening with your beta cells. They're not renewable resources—once they're gone, they're gone for good. So, if you're not taking care of them now (we'll discuss how to protect these valuable assets in the next chapter), you're essentially spending your health savings before you even know its value. Are you ready to start protecting your beta cell piggy bank and treating them with the respect they deserve? Because trust me, your future self will thank you for every cell you save today.

Here's the shocking reality: By the time you're officially labeled "prediabetic," you've already lost about half of your precious insulin-producing beta cells. Half! It's like waking up one day to find that half your life savings has vanished overnight. If you wait until you are diagnosed with "diabetes," up to 80% of your beta cells could be depleted! And here's the gut-punch—those cells aren't coming back. Once they're gone, they're gone for good. It's like trying to run a marathon on one leg—possible, but why make it harder on yourself?

These aren't just statistics; it's a WAKE-UP CALL. Every day you wait, you're losing more of these vital cells: a chance to turn things around, to protect what you have left, and to rewrite your health story. The power is in your hands, but the clock is ticking. Are you ready to take action before it's too late?

Here's the game-changer: we don't have to fight a losing battle. About 98 million Americans have prediabetes, but more than 8 in 10 adults don't know they have it [Source: Prediabetes: Could It Be You? Infographic]. If you and I spread the word on early diagnosis and prevention, we could be on the brink of a health revolution.

Right now, you have a golden opportunity to shield your remaining beta cells and potentially undo some of the damage. But what if I told you there's a way to spot trouble years before standard tests can? This isn't sci-fi or some exclusive test only for the uber wealthy. It's a powerful tool that's been right under our noses, yet tragically underused. Chances are, no one's ever ordered this test for you. But today, that changes. You're about to unlock a secret weapon in your health arsenal—one that could rewrite your entire health story. Are you ready to take control and glimpse into your metabolic future?

Here is the **secret weapon**: a fasting insulin blood draw. It's the test that only 1% of healthcare providers order routinely, but it can identify 80% of people affected with prediabetes. It's like having a crystal ball that can see 13 years into your metabolic future.

The next time you visit your health care provider, ask for a fasting insulin test. Knowing your insulin level is the difference between stumbling through life hoping for the best and confidently steering your health in the right direction. By keeping your insulin well below 9, you're not just preventing diabetes—you're optimizing your metabolism, sharpening your focus, and building a body primed for longevity and performance. This isn't just survival—it's strategic, science-backed thriving.

Remember, this isn't about fear—it's about arming yourself with knowledge. You hold the power to rewrite your health story. Knowing the signs and symptoms of diabetes AND proactive screening, utilizing early detection tools like insulin, are the keys to unlocking a life where diabetes isn't even on your radar. It's your chance to act with purpose—not play defense. Don't wait for problems to show up—get ahead of the game and start living the Type Zero life today.

Now that you're armed with the knowledge to stay ahead of diabetes, it's time to tackle the next crucial piece of the puzzle: fueling your body with the right nutrition. Because when it comes to taking control, what you put on your plate is your most powerful prescription.

CHAPTER 3

Fork Your Way to Freedom: Nutrition as Your New Prescription

"The doctor of the future will give no medicine, but will interest his patient in the care of the human frame, in diet and in the cause and prevention of disease."
— Thomas Edison (1903)

As an endocrinologist who faced and reversed her own prediabetes diagnosis, I'm here to tell you that managing your blood sugar does not mean zero pleasures or indulgences. No drastic fasting, no questionable detoxes, and certainly no fad diets. Instead, I want to show you my Type Zero nutrition prescription—a sustainable approach that's both effective and enjoyable.

The Power of Breakfast & Balanced Plates

"Breakfast is everything. The beginning, the first thing. It is the mouthful that is the commitment to a new day."
— A. A. Gill

I have heard so many people tell me, "But I'm not hungry in the morning." If that is you, let me break it down to you. You are not hungry in the morning because your body has gotten used to the routine of eating later in the day, and your metabolism has slowed down or is in a deep hibernation. The two best ways to reset your metabolism are to finish eating earlier at night (yes, I'm calling out all of you night owls who are snacking on popcorn while watching your Netflix show at 11 p.m.) and start having SOMEthing for breakfast, even if it's just a couple of bites.

Numerous studies have shown that eating breakfast can significantly lower your risk of developing type 2 diabetes and metabolic syndrome compared to skipping it altogether. When you eat breakfast, it has a positive impact on how your body handles carbohydrates. This means that your body is better at using insulin in the morning (insulin sensitivity), which is important for keeping your blood sugar levels under control all day long.

High-fiber, high-protein breakfasts are winners when it comes to stabilizing your blood sugar levels and boosting your insulin sensitivity. Think of it as setting your body up for success right from the morning. Simply putting something nutritious in your belly in the morning, especially a macro-balanced meal, is linked to a lower risk of type 2 diabetes.

So, make sure you're not skipping out on this crucial meal!

I usually rotate between these breakfast meals:

- A coffee protein shake (I mix coffee, protein powder, and almond milk together and no longer need creamer or sugar for my coffee!)

- Greek yogurt topped with berries and walnuts (skip the granola to avoid hidden sugars)
- One slice of thin-cut whole grain bread (like Dave's Killer Bread) topped with avocado or light Laughing Cow cheese, spinach, and an egg

These options provide a balanced start to my day, combining protein, healthy fats, and complex carbohydrates to keep my blood sugar stable, my energy high, and my metabolism supercharged.

For lunch and dinner, I have adopted a simple yet powerful strategy: the 40-40-20 plate. That's 40% lean protein, 40% vegetables, and 20% whole grain carbs (my simple definition of a whole grain carb is that it has at least 3 g of fiber per healthy serving). This approach not only makes my meals visually appealing and satisfying, but it also provides me with the nutrients I need for sustained energy and mental focus until my next meal or snack.

Lean Proteins: Your Metabolic Powerhouse

Protein takes the most energy to break down and use by your body compared to other types of nutrients. This process, called the thermic effect of food, can boost your metabolism by using 20–30% of the calories from the protein you eat. For instance, if you consume 100 calories of protein, your body might only use 70 of those calories because it burns the other 30 calories during the digestion and processing process.

In comparison, carbohydrates use 5–15% of their energy for digestion, with complex carbs using more than simple or processed ones. Fats use the least energy, only 0–5%, because they are easy to digest.

Just to amplify this point again, protein has the highest thermic effect, followed by carbs, then fats. This makes protein excellent for weight management and metabolic health because it uses a lot of energy to digest and helps keep you full and maintain muscle. Lean proteins are also crucial for blood sugar management. They help slow digestion, promoting fullness and reducing glucose spikes. Opt for sources like:

- Skinless poultry
- Fish
- Turkey
- Tofu
- Low-fat dairy
- Eggs

Research shows that incorporating these protein sources can lower your risk of type 2 diabetes by up to 35%!

Vegetables: Nature's Medicine

Vegetables are your secret weapon in the fight against diabetes. Veggies are high in fiber, which helps your body digest food slowly. This keeps your blood sugar levels stable and can even reduce the risk of type 2 diabetes. They are also full of vitamins A, C, and E, which help reduce inflammation and may lower the risk of diabetes complications. Finally, veggies like arugula and celery are rich in nitrates, which can help lower blood pressure and reduce the risk of heart disease, two diseases often linked to diabetes, creating the Metabolic Syndrome.

When managing diabetes, it is important to be mindful of the sugar and carbohydrate content of the vegetables you consume. Here are some of the sweeter and higher-carbohydrate vegetables that should be eaten in moderation [Source 1]:

- Sweet Potatoes: Contain up to 5.5% sugar
- Beets: Contain up to 8% sugar
- Sweet Corn: Contains up to 6.3% sugar
- Green Peas: Contain up to 5.9% sugar
- Carrots: While not as high in sugar as some others, they still contain up to 4.7% sugar
- Winter Squash and Butternut Squash: These are high in carbohydrates and should be consumed in moderation

Aim to fill nearly 40% of your plate with non-starchy vegetables, such as leafy greens, broccoli, cauliflower, and bell peppers. While some vegetables, like sweet potatoes (up to 5.5 g of sugar per 100 g), beets (up to 8 g per 100 g), and sweet corn (up to 6.3 g per 100 g), have higher sugar content, they still contain less sugar than most fruits, which I will discuss next.

Fruit: Nature's Candy in Moderation

This is definitely where I hear wailing and moaning. My patients ask, "How can fruit be unhealthy?" Yes, fruits are nutritious, but they do contain natural sugars and often have a much higher sugar content than vegetables. For example, apples contain about 11.1 g of sugar per 100 g, bananas have around 12.8 g per 100 g, and pineapples have approximately 8.2 g per 100 g.

An interesting study led by Harvard School of Public Health found that eating at least two servings per week of whole fruits like blueberries, grapes, and apples reduced the risk of type 2 diabetes by up to 23%

compared to those who ate less than one serving per month [Source 2]. Whole fruits are packed with fiber (which slows sugar absorption and keeps blood sugar steady), loaded with antioxidants (to fight inflammation and help your body use insulin better), and great for your gut health (which also supports healthy blood sugar levels).

But even with all these benefits, it's smart to watch your portions— eating too much fruit can still add up to a lot of natural sugar, which may raise your diabetes risk if you go overboard. Moderation is key!

When it comes to stabilizing blood sugar, some fruits are better than others due to their low glycemic index, high fiber, and beneficial polyphenols and antioxidants. Here are the top picks: berries, oranges, grapefruits, apples, pears, and peaches. And to help you enjoy them without the sugar spike, here's the Dr. Hormone Hacker Guideline for smart, healthy fruit portions.

- Small fruits like grapes, cherries: ten
- Small fruits like tangerines, plums, apricots: one
- Medium fruits like apples, peaches, pears, oranges: half of the fruit
- Berries: ½ cup
- Melons: 4–5 pieces in a cut-up bowl you would see at the grocery store/restaurant

The Best Order for Eating Macros

Did you know that the order in which you consume proteins, vegetables, and carbohydrates is significant for your blood sugars? I certainly didn't, until I dove into the research. A study from Weill Cornell Medical College found that when patients with type 2 diabetes and obesity ate vegetables and protein before carbohydrates, their glucose levels were 29%, 37%, and 17% lower at 30, 60, and 120 minutes after the meal, respectively, compared to eating carbohydrates first [Source 3].

So, here is the game plan when you sit down for a meal:

1. Start your meal with non-starchy vegetables high in fiber and low in calories (broccoli, spinach). Eating these first slows down how quickly the rest of your food digests, which reduces the sudden spike in your blood sugar levels. When you are at a restaurant, go for the side salad before your meal, but I double dare you to skip the bread or tortilla chip basket!

2. Follow with protein, which takes longer to digest than carbohydrates, which helps in slowing down the absorption of glucose into the bloodstream.

3. Save the carbs, especially the refined or high-glycemic ones like bread, rice, and pasta, for last. When you are at an asian restaurant, don't order fried rice, where the rice is already mixed in and it's hard to separate out the vegetables and protein. Order something where the rice or noodles are on the side so YOU get to decide WHEN to eat them. By doing this, the fiber and protein from the earlier parts of your meal can slow down how quickly the carbs are digested and absorbed. This helps keep your blood sugar and insulin levels from spiking too high.

Not All Protein Bars Are Created Equal

Many people often reach for protein bars or granola bars, thinking they are making a healthy snack choice, but many are glorified candy bars. These bars, while convenient and appearing wholesome, can be loaded with carbs and sugar that can spike sugar levels. For instance, a typical granola bar can contain anywhere from 13 to 23 grams of carbs and 7 to 13 grams of sugar, as seen with products like Larabar and Quaker Chewy Dipps.

To illustrate this point, let's consider a specific example: a Clif Bar. A single serving of a Clif Bar can contain up to 43 grams of carbs, which is comparable to the amount found in a medium order of fries at a fast food restaurant. Additionally, it includes 17 grams of sugar, equivalent to the amount in an apple fritter. This is a significant amount, especially if you're watching your sugar intake. I tell people you should only be consuming such a bar if you're about to climb a big cliff—hence the name!

For everyday snacking, it's crucial to check the ingredient labels and opt for bars that are made from whole foods, have less than 17 grams of net carbs (carbs minus fiber), at least 2 grams of fiber (the higher, the better), less than 9 grams of fat, and 20-plus grams of protein to keep you full and satisfied without the unwanted sugar and carb overload. Two of my favorites are Pure Protein and Quest bars.

The Oatmeal Myth

Many of my patients proudly declared they were eating oatmeal to lower their cholesterol. My response? "By the time you lower your cholesterol eating that much oatmeal, you might give yourself diabetes!" A serving of flavored oatmeal with raisins and bananas typically contains around 30–40 grams of carbohydrates and 10–15 grams of sugar.

It's often seen as a super healthy breakfast, but here's the thing—it can actually give you a surprise sugar spike if you're not careful. Don't worry, though, you can still enjoy your morning bowl with the following Dr. Hormone Hacker tweaks.

Start by skipping the instant flavored packets and go for hearty steel-cut or rolled oats instead—you can level it up even more by choosing a protein-packed option like Kodiak to turn your breakfast into a performance meal.

Use either water or 30-calorie unsweetened almond milk for the liquid. And portion size matters—stick to about half a cup of dry oats.

Now, the fun part—toppings! Skip the sugary stuff and try these instead:

- A small handful of almonds or walnuts (about 7–8)
- Some unsweetened coconut flakes (2 tablespoons)
- A sprinkle of flax seeds
- A few berries instead of a banana. Here's a cool trick: freeze some blueberries and toss about ¼ cup into your oatmeal while it's cooking. It's like a natural sweetener, but healthier.

Fun fact: freezing blueberries makes them taste sweeter! The water inside expands when frozen, bursting the cells and releasing more natural sugars. So, you get extra sweetness without adding any sugar.

Now, you know how to hack oatmeal so it works for you, not against you. These topping options will add flavor and nutrition without the sugar overload. Plus, they'll keep you feeling full and energized instead of tired and sleepy after the sugar crash.

Sweet Deception: The Truth About Acai Bowls and Smoothies

One word: ABORT! Acai bowls might seem like a health food paradise, but they're often sugar bombs in disguise. An average acai bowl can contain up to 50–75 grams of sugar and 100 grams of carbohydrates. That's like eating 3–4 candy bars in one sitting!

Here's the truth about acai bowls: the berries themselves are actually low in sugar, but those toppings and sweeteners are where the sugar bomb comes from. But don't write them off just yet! Acai is packed with antioxidants—we're talking 10 to 30 times more than strawberries. Pretty impressive, right? Oh, and here's a fun tidbit: these berries go bad super fast, like within 24 hours of picking. That's why you usually see them frozen or powdered. So, if you're craving an acai bowl, maybe share one with a friend or whip up your own at home. That way, you can control the sugar while still getting those awesome antioxidants.

Like acai bowls, smoothies can be carbohydrate heavyweights. A typical 20-ounce smoothie can contain 70–80 grams of carbs and 50–60 grams of sugar. If you enjoy smoothies, make them at home where you can control the ingredients. Focus on vegetables (especially green ones like spinach, kale, and cucumber), a small amount of fruit (refer to my fruit portions guideline above), and add protein powder or Greek yogurt for balance. By being savvy with your smoothie-making, you can whip up a drink that's both delicious and healthy to create a smart snack, not a deceptive sugar bomb.

Flavor Boosters or Sugar Bombs? The Condiment Catch-22

I need to expose some sneaky sugar sources that often fly under the radar. Condiments can be silent saboteurs of your blood sugar goals. Many popular sauces are loaded with hidden sugars:

- BBQ sauce: Often contains up to 13 g of sugar per 2 tablespoons
- Ketchup: About 4 g of sugar per tablespoon
- Spaghetti sauce: Can have up to 12 g of sugar per half-cup serving
- Sweet chili sauce: Has nearly 14 grams in 2 tablespoons
- Ken's Steakhouse Country French with Orange Blossom Honey: 9 grams of sugar in 2 tablespoons, which is nearly equal to adding 2 teaspoons of pure sugar on your salad!

And let's talk about portion sizes, shall we? When was the last time you actually whipped out a measuring spoon for your ketchup? Yeah, I thought so. Those labels suggesting a "serving size" of one or two tablespoons are living in a fantasy world where people delicately dab condiments onto their food like they're painting a Monet.

In reality, most of us are more Jackson Pollock with our sauces, creating abstract expressionist masterpieces on our plates. And don't even get me started on BBQ sauce—that's not a condiment, it's a lifestyle choice.

So, while you're busy turning your burger into a sugary, saucy Slip 'N Slide, you could be unknowingly doubling or tripling your sugar intake. So, what can we do? Here are some ways to hack these sugary pitfalls:

- Opt for **low-sugar** or **no-sugar-added** versions of your favorite condiments. Brands like Rao's for pasta sauce or reduced-sugar ketchup options are great alternatives.
- Try making your own sauces at home. A homemade tomato sauce or salad dressing can be just as flavorful without the added sugars.
- Pay attention to ingredient labels. Sugar can hide under names like dextrose, fructose, high-fructose corn syrup, and maltose.

By being mindful of these sneaky sources, you can enjoy your favorite condiments without derailing your health goals!

Ditching the Sweet Sips

Let's talk about what really happens when you pop open that soda or sip that sugary iced tea. You're not just enjoying a refreshing drink— you're sending your body into a sugar frenzy.

With each gulp, your blood glucose levels skyrocket, and your poor pancreas goes into panic mode, pumping out insulin to manage the surge. It's not just a momentary sugar high; it's a metabolic rollercoaster that can have serious long-term consequences.

Consider this: drinking just 1–2 sugary beverages daily increases your risk of developing type 2 diabetes by 26% compared to those who rarely indulge [Source 4]. And let's not forget about those "empty calories." A single can of cola packs about 39 grams of sugar—that's already more than the American Heart Association recommends for your entire DAY (for men: no more than 36 grams/9 teaspoons daily; for women: no more than 25 grams/6 teaspoons daily)! You're essentially drinking your way to potential weight gain and health issues, one sweet sip at a time.

Remember, sugar-sweetened beverages (SSBs) are not just sodas; they also include: fruit drinks, sports drinks, energy drinks, coffee drinks, and electrolyte replacement drinks. When you look at the nutritional label for a drink, **keep it less than 7 grams** of carbs and sugar, the lower the better!

This study caught my attention: a group of overweight teens was put through a mini sugar detox, and the results were eye-opening. After just three days without their beloved sugary drinks, these kids were a mess. We're talking full-blown withdrawal symptoms: intense cravings, throbbing headaches, and decreased motivation, contentment, ability to concentrate, and overall well-being [Source 5]. We have known for years about the effects of caffeine withdrawal, but now we're seeing the impact of raising a generation of sugar junkies.

Now, let's connect the dots. If teens are kickstarting their days with what's essentially a sugar bomb, is it any wonder that obesity and diabetes rates are going through the roof? The numbers are staggering:

- Nearly 1 in 5 American kids aged 2–19 are obese. There is no data on how many kids in this age group are overweight, but it could be 3 in 5 teens!
- Type 2 diabetes in youth? It's skyrocketed by a whopping 95% in the last two decades.
- On average, teens are gulping down about 143 calories from sugary drinks every single day.

It's like we're unwittingly raising a generation of sugar addicts. If a few days without it can cause such havoc, what's it doing to our kids over the next several years or decades?

If you are 12 to 19 years old, your rate of prediabetes has more than doubled between 1999 and 2002 and between 2015 and 2018, jumping from 12% to 28%! Nearly one in three adolescents and teens now has prediabetes. Imagine being barely old enough to drive, and you've just signed up for a 50-plus-year marathon of dodging diabetes bullets along with heart disease, kidney problems, and liver disease. So, before you reach for that next sugary sip, ask yourself: *Is a moment of sweetness worth sacrificing decades of health?*

But here's the good news: You don't have to go cold turkey overnight. Think of it as a gradual lifestyle shift rather than an all-or-nothing challenge. Start small—try swapping out just one sugary drink a day for a healthier alternative. Maybe replace that mid-afternoon soda with a sparkling water (I love refreshing citrus-flavored ones like tangerine, grapefruit, or lime) or experiment with unsweetened iced tea (I add strawberry or orange slices in mine).

Start making the switch TODAY. As you get comfortable with this change, slowly increase your swaps. Your future self will thank you for every soda you skip and every glass of water you choose. Let's raise a glass (of water, of course) to your health!

Brewing Danger: The Dark Side of Sweetened Coffee

Picture this: You're innocently sipping on what you think is a harmless cup of joe, when in reality, you could be drinking your way to diabetes. That grande pumpkin spice latte you're clutching? It's not just warming your hands; it's also dumping a whopping 50 grams of sugar into your unsuspecting body. So, before you take another sip, ask yourself: Is this just coffee, or dessert in a cup?

Now, I know what you're thinking: *But this is the ONE thing I enjoy each morning and it's sacred.* These drinks are engineered to delight our taste buds and keep us coming back for more. It's like they've cracked the code to our sugar-loving souls, and they have, because it has been shown that both sugar and caffeine have addictive properties.

So, what's a coffee lover to do? Let me offer you some healthy hacks:

1. **Play barista bartender**: Add a splash of hot water to your brew. It softens the acidity of the coffee, thereby requiring fewer sweeteners.

2. **Bean there, done that**: Flavored coffee beans, like vanilla or hazelnut, can give you that hint of sweetness without any added sugar.

3. **Spice up your life**: Sprinkle in some cinnamon, nutmeg, or even cocoa powder for a natural flavor boost.

4. **Milk it for all it's worth**: Switch to unsweetened almond or coconut milk. They're naturally sweeter and can help cut down on added sweeteners. Oat and soy milk have slightly higher carbohydrate content, but still relatively low sugar levels when unsweetened. Cow's milk has about 4–12 times more carbs and 6–12 times more sugar than unsweetened almond milk, but it does have more protein.

5. **Extract some flavor**: A drop of vanilla or almond extract goes a long way and can work wonders for flavor without the sugar.

6. **Play coffee roulette**: If you're a multiple-cup-a-day person, try making every other cup unsweetened to ease into the habit.

7. **Size does matter**: Use a smaller cup. It's not downsizing, it's "right-sizing" your coffee experience.

8. **Keep your cool**: Try cold brew. It's naturally smoother and less bitter, so you might not need as much sweetness to enjoy it.

9. **My protein-packed coffee hack**: I add a scoop of chocolate protein powder to my coffee and make an iced coffee protein shake; that way, I don't have to add any cream or sugar at all, it tastes like an iced cafe mocha, and I start my day with 25 g of protein.

10. **Perk-fection: Optimizing your caffeine fuel**: I've cracked the code for smooth, all-day energy. My secret? Aromatic teas like Earl Grey. A splash of unsweetened almond milk is all I need—no sugar crashes here. It's my go-to for steady caffeine without the heart-racing drama.

Remember, cutting back on sweeteners is a journey, not a sprint. Your taste buds might throw a little tantrum at first, but they'll thank you later. Now, let's tackle the controversial elephant in the room: the pros and cons of artificial sweeteners.

The Sweet Debate: Decoding Your Colorful Sweetener Options

Before you reach for that rainbow of sweetener packets at your local coffee shop, let's take a moment to decode the colorful world of artificial sweeteners. You know the ones I'm talking about—pink, blue, green, yellow—they're like a sugar-free Skittles lineup.

Let's break down what's really in those packets.

First, artificial sweeteners range from 200 to 700 times sweeter than table sugar, while some can be up to 13,000 times sweeter than sugar

[Source 6]. Imagine what that does to your taste buds—no wonder people who drink diet sodas don't typically like the taste of water. Artificial sweeteners may overstimulate sugar receptors, which can make foods that are not intensely sweet (fruits and vegetables) less appealing.

Second, when comparing Sweet'N Low (saccharin), Equal (aspartame), and stevia-based sweeteners like Truvia in relation to diabetes risk, a large study looked at over 100,000 people and found some startling results. People who regularly reached for the sweet stuff without the calories had a higher chance of developing type 2 diabetes compared to those who didn't use these sweeteners at all [Source 7].

Finally, artificial sweeteners can act like the ultimate tricksters of the food world. These cheeky little molecules are like that friend who promises an epic night out but shows up in pajamas with a bowl of popcorn, asking which movie you're watching on Netflix. It's as if your body is all dressed up for a calorie party, only to find out it's been punk'd. They activate the sweet taste receptors but don't provide the calories our bodies expect. Imagine biting into a juicy apple, but it tastes like cotton candy. Some research suggests this sweet deception might backfire. Your brain, expecting a calorie boost that never comes, might hit the hunger alarm [Source 8]. It's like your body's saying, "Hey, you promised me energy! Where is it?" This confusion could lead you to munch more—the ultimate metabolic bait-and-switch!

What does this mean for you? Well, it looks like those "healthier" sugar alternatives might not be the magic bullet for avoiding diabetes that we once thought. In fact, they might be doing more harm than good when it comes to preventing diabetes. Here is what I do: if I am sweetening my coffee or tea, I reach for a green or yellow packet and use no more than ¼ of the packet—yes, only ¼. There is no definitive proven amount that is safe, so wean yourself down to the smallest amount possible.

But hold onto your forks and coffee spoons! While we've been dissecting our diets, we've only uncovered half the secret sauce in our diabetes-busting recipe. Now, it's time to push away from the table (just a little) and trade in your fork for some dumbbells. In our next chapter, we'll explore why those tiny beads of perspiration are actually your body's way of shedding more than just water. It's time to turn up the burn on diabetes prevention!

CHAPTER 4

Sweat Is Just Fat Crying: The Sweet Science of Exercise

"My favorite machine at the gym is the television."
— Unknown

Hey, whatever gets you through those last ten minutes on the treadmill. I'm not here to judge.

As an endocrinologist, I used to preach the gospel of cardio like it was the holy grail of diabetes prevention. "Just hop on that treadmill for 30 minutes a day," I'd say, secretly dreading my own monotonous jogs on the treadmill. I was sprinting on a glucose-fueled treadmill, racing against my own biology to outpace prediabetes. Spoiler alert: It wasn't working. This hamster on a never-ending wheel needed to change the game and build her muscles, not just tone her legs. Who knew that the key to glucose control was less about running in circles and more about pumping some iron?

Ah, the dreaded "E" word: exercise. It's enough to make some of us break out in a cold sweat—and not the good kind from a workout! Let's face it, when you hear "exercise," your brain might instantly conjure up emotions such as hate, dread, fear, and guilt.

As an endocrinologist, I've heard every excuse in the book for avoiding exercise. From "the treadmill is so boring" to "I get injured or I'm sore for weeks after exercise." I get it—time is scarce, and the "runner's high" feels more like a cruel myth. But here's the sugar-free truth: Your pancreas is begging you to move.

Exercise isn't just about slipping into those perfectly fitted jeans, though that's definitely a sweet perk! Think of regular workouts as giving your body a smart upgrade to help prevent or improve diabetes. When you break a sweat, you're not just burning calories. Suddenly, your muscles develop an intelligent algorithm for sucking up excess sugar from your bloodstream more efficiently. It's like upgrading your metabolism from a clunky flip phone to the latest smartphone—everything just runs smoother, faster, and more efficiently.

Imagine your body's cells have tiny doors that let sugar in, and insulin is the key that unlocks these doors. For people with prediabetes or diabetes, these doors get rusty over time, making it harder for insulin to do its job. That's where exercise comes in, like a magical WD-40 for your cellular doors!

When you do a moderate workout—think of a brisk walk that leaves you a little breathless but still able to chat—something amazing happens within 15 minutes of starting your workout. Your body's cells suddenly become 51% better at responding to insulin [Source 9]. If you're feeling ambitious, high-intensity exercise (a 20-minute rowing session) cranks that up to a whopping 85%. If you need even more motivation, a study in the *British Journal of Sports Medicine* found that people who engaged in moderate to vigorous exercise for up to an hour a day had a whopping 74% lower risk of developing type 2 diabetes. That's a life-changing return on a small daily investment!

And here's the best part—exercise can improve your insulin sensitivity for up to 48 hours after you're done [Source 10]. That's right, your body keeps reaping the benefits long after you've hit the showers.

Now that you know the importance of exercise in combating diabetes, it's time to transform that knowledge into action. The question isn't about finding time—it's about PRIORITIZING time for what truly matters: your long-term health.

Staying active while traveling or during a busy day can be challenging, but with a few simple tricks, you can incorporate more movement into your routine without disrupting your schedule. Here are some of my favorite hacks to keep you energized and moving throughout the day:

- I pack my resistance bands when I'm on vacation. They're incredibly lightweight and easy to roll up into my tennis shoes, making them the perfect travel companion for quick workouts anywhere. This way, I can maintain my strength training routine even when I'm away from home.
- When that mid-afternoon slump hits, instead of reaching for another cup of coffee (which could be my second or third!), I opt for a quick five-minute session of jumping jacks, squats, and planks. It's amazing how these simple exercises instantly perk me up and get my blood flowing, providing a natural energy boost without the caffeine crash.
- During TV commercials, especially while watching sporting events, I do some chair yoga. It's a great way to stretch and relax without missing any of the action on screen.

Here are seven additional practical and easy ideas to naturally incorporate more movement into your day:

1. **Phone Pacing**: When I'm on a phone call, I pace around my room or house. It's an effortless way to add steps to my day.

2. **Desk Stretches**: Set a timer to remind yourself to do some simple stretches at your desk every hour. Shoulder rolls, neck rotations, and seated twists can help improve circulation and reduce stiffness.

3. **Stair Challenge**: If you work in a building with stairs, challenge yourself to use them instead of the elevator at least once a day. It's a great way to get your heart rate up.

4. **Walking Meetings**: Suggest walking meetings for one-on-one discussions with colleagues. It's a refreshing change of pace and allows you to get some steps in while being productive.

5. **Commercial Break Challenges**: During longer TV sessions, set yourself mini-challenges during commercial breaks. Try to do as many push-ups, lunges, or arm circles (remember those from middle school PE class?!) as you can before your show resumes.

6. **Hydration Walks**: Every time you need to refill your water bottle, take a longer route to the water cooler or kitchen. It's an easy way to add more steps and stay hydrated.

7. **Lunge While You Brush**: Turn daily routines into movement opportunities! While brushing your teeth, do a set of walking lunges or hold a wall sit. It's a simple way to sneak in strength work during tasks you're already doing—no extra time required.

By incorporating these simple activities into your daily routine, you can significantly increase your overall movement without feeling like you're sacrificing time or energy. Remember, every little bit counts when it comes to staying active and healthy!

Now that you know how to add more simple and efficient movement into your day, your ultimate mission is to clock in 150 minutes of moderate-intensity aerobic activity each week. That's similar to watching a full-length Marvel movie while jogging in place—except this time, you're the one taking charge of your metabolism like a true superhero.

Here's your game plan:

- Spread those 150 minutes over at least 3 days. Your body loves consistency more than your ex loves your social media posts.
- If you're feeling spicy, trade in those 150 moderate minutes for 75 vigorous ones. It's like speed dating, but for your health.
- Don't ghost your workout routine for more than 2 days in a row. Your cells get separation anxiety.

Mix it up with brisk walks, cycling, or swimming. Or try HIIT—it's like espresso shots for your insulin sensitivity. Throw in some resistance training, too; your muscles and glucose levels will high-five you for it.

Remember, even small steps count. Start with 10–15 minutes a day and build up. Your body will thank you by potentially keeping diabetes at bay. It's like compound interest for your health!

For people who are not able to walk, consider refreshing pool exercises or chair yoga. Starting an exercise routine doesn't mean you have to become a gym rat overnight. Begin with small, achievable goals. Maybe it's a 10-minute walk after dinner or a few strength exercises during commercial breaks.

By gradually increasing the intensity of your workouts, you're not just building strength and endurance—you're sculpting a leaner you because exercise is your superpower against visceral fat.

What is visceral fat, and why is it such a problem? This is the fat that surrounds your internal organs. VAT (visceral adipose tissue) actively interferes with your body's insulin response, essentially creating a "no-entry" zone for insulin to do its job of regulating blood sugar [Source 11].

Here's the surprising plot twist in the world of diabetes research: for years, we've been pointing fingers at obesity as the big bad wolf of type 2 diabetes. But recent studies have revealed a surprising new villain in the diabetes story: VAT [Source 12].

This game-changing discovery turns our understanding of type 2 diabetes risk factors on its head. It's not just about how much you weigh, but WHERE your body stores its fat. Someone with a higher BMI but less VAT might actually be at lower risk than someone with a "normal" BMI but more VAT. It's like we've been focused on the tip of the iceberg, only to realize the real danger lurks beneath the surface.

The good news? Targeted exercises and dietary changes can help reduce VAT, potentially lowering your T2D risk more effectively than focusing solely on overall weight loss. For example, when someone is taking a medication like Ozempic, they may be losing weight on the scale, but it would be more significant to see how much visceral fat is being lost and how much muscle is being maintained or increased. It's a reminder that when it comes to health, what's happening beneath the surface often matters more than what we see on the scale.

If you're looking to wage war on VAT, recent research has uncovered some heavy hitters in the fight against this internal troublemaker. Let's dive into the best exercises:

Aerobic Exercise: The VAT Vanquisher

Aerobic exercise, especially when it's cranked up to vigorous intensity, is your secret weapon against VAT. Some top-notch options include:

- Brisk walking (pick up the pace, folks!)
- Running (invest in a pair of shoes that'll make your feet float and your VAT weep)
- Swimming (make a splash against VAT)
- Cycling (pedal your way to a leaner you)

HIIT: The VAT Blaster

High-Intensity Interval Training (HIIT) is like a lightning strike to your VAT. It's quick, it's intense, and it gets the job done. Some HIIT exercises to try:

- Burpees (the exercise everyone loves to hate)
- Mountain climbers (scaling your way to less VAT)
- Jump squats (hop to it for better health)

Resistance Training: The Unexpected Hero

Don't count out strength training in your battle against VAT! Resistance training flexes its VAT-busting muscles especially for:

- Males (sorry, ladies, this one's more effective for the guys) [Source 13]
- People with body fat percentage under 40% (less cushion, more VAT-crushing)

The Dynamic Duo: Aerobic + Resistance

Why choose when you can have both? Combining aerobic exercise with resistance training is like assembling your own personal VAT-fighting squad. It's a one-two punch that leaves visceral fat reeling. Remember, consistency is key. These exercises aren't magic pills—they're more like daily vitamins for your metabolism.

Pro tip: While vigorous aerobic exercise and HIIT seem to be the heavyweight champs in the VAT-busting arena, the best exercise is the one you'll actually do. So find something you enjoy, crank up the intensity when you can, and get moving!

I now channel my inner kid (minus the ability to eat junk food without consequences) and make exercise fun again. I'm out there trying to master pickleball (it's like tennis for people who don't want to run as much), attending hip-hop classes (often making my kids cringe), and even doing a Pilates video on YouTube (because sometimes, leaving the house is overrated).

So, I encourage you to diversify your exercise routine. Mix it up and have fun. Whether it's joining a local sports league, taking a dance class, or just doing some resistance band exercises while binge-watching your favorite show, find what works for you.

The question remains:

- Do you prefer your remedy in reps or recipes?
- Your cure in curls or capsules?
- Your therapy in deadlifts or doses?
- So, what'll it be?
- Bench-press your way to better health,

- Or let a pill do the heavy lifting?

As you embark on your fitness journey, keep in mind that every drop of sweat is a deposit in the bank of longevity. Now, if you'll excuse me, I have a date with some dumbbells and a YouTube video promising to give me abs of steel.

But as much as we love those post-workout endorphins, the real game-changer in your health journey isn't just about what you do in the gym—it's also about what happens when you're not working out. Let's talk about how stress and sleepless nights are silently sabotaging your blood sugar, and why it's time to take control of your rest.

CHAPTER 5

Sleepless and Stressed: Your Blood Sugar's Worst Nightmare

"I finally got eight hours of sleep. It took me three days, but whatever." — Unknown

Sleep and stress—those subtle manipulators—have a tendency to disrupt your blood sugar levels without drawing attention. This chapter spills the tea on how these two can crash the party and throw your glucose levels into chaos, transforming your body's smooth rhythm into total mayhem.

Let's start with the basics: sleep is not just for drooling on your pillow anymore, or dreaming about landing your dream job, or finally mastering that tricky yoga pose. It's a crucial period when your body performs a range of metabolic functions that keep your blood sugar levels in check. During sleep, especially in those deep, restorative stages, your body works the graveyard shift to regulate insulin sensitivity and glucose metabolism. This nocturnal process is far more than just a nightly recharge—your body is actually doing an "Extreme Makeover: Hormone Edition."

Research shows that your glucose levels can actually get a little adventurous during a good night's sleep, rising by as much as 20% before they settle back down by morning [Source 14]. But here's the kicker: if you're slacking on sleep, that careful balancing act gets thrown off course. It's like trying to navigate a road trip with a GPS that keeps recalculating—you think your glucose levels are on track, but insulin's guidance system starts malfunctioning, and things can veer off course faster than you'd expect.

Studies suggest that just ONE night of poor sleep can mess with insulin's ability to do its job, making your body more insulin-resistant and less tolerant to glucose, leading to temporary pre-diabetic conditions [Source 15].

I used to burn the midnight oil, working long past midnight, because that was when the house was finally quiet and the kids were in bed (anyone else treasure those peaceful nocturnal moments?). However, that late-night productivity came with a price.

I also remember how I'd feel the next day after staying up late to binge-watch TV. We've all been there—the sluggish, zombie-like start to the day that makes you feel like you're wading through molasses. But what I didn't realize at the time was that these "harmless" late-night habits were actually nudging my body toward a pre-diabetic state.

Now, that's what happens with just ONE night of not getting enough sleep. But let's be real—how easy is it to slip into a pattern where this becomes the new norm? A groundbreaking study revealed that just one week of sleep restriction (as in, only five hours per night) led to a shocking 30% reduction in insulin sensitivity—an effect that mirrored what you'd typically see in individuals already living with type 2 diabetes [Source 14].

When we talk about "good quality sleep," it's more than just hitting the pillow for a solid 7–9 hours. What really matters is getting enough time in the deep, restorative stages of sleep, specifically the slow-wave and REM stages. These are the phases where your body isn't just resting: insulin helps cells absorb glucose efficiently, cortisol keeps stress in check, and growth hormone promotes tissue repair. When all these hormones are in sync, your body is better equipped to prevent insulin resistance, process glucose efficiently, and recover for the day ahead.

Two other hormones—ghrelin and leptin—play key roles in keeping your blood sugar in check. Ghrelin, known as the "hunger hormone," signals your brain when to eat, while leptin, the "satiety hormone," tells you when you're full. When you don't get enough quality sleep, ghrelin levels go up, making you feel hungrier, and leptin levels drop, leaving you less satisfied after meals. This imbalance can lead to overeating, weight gain, and, eventually, insulin resistance.

Who knew that even estrogen and testosterone levels are affected by sleep quality? For women, poor sleep isn't just a beauty issue—it's a metabolic one. Estrogen, which helps regulate insulin sensitivity, takes a hit when we don't get enough rest. The result? Insulin resistance rises, making it a whole lot harder to button our jeans and keep blood sugar in check. For men, the sleep struggle is just as real. When you skimp on sleep, your testosterone levels drop, triggering fat storage (especially around the belly) and blood sugar spikes. So, no matter how much you crush it at the gym or try to eat clean, your body won't cooperate when it comes to managing glucose.

But don't worry, there's good news—getting your hormones back on track isn't as complicated as it sounds. The keys? Sleep timing and consistency. Yep, the when of sleep matters just as much as the how much. Research shows that going to bed and waking up at the same time every day helps to synchronize your circadian rhythm, which helps regulate these crucial hormones [Source 16]. But it's not just about getting enough sleep—it's all about what time you hit the sack.

Imagine this: You're wide awake at 2 a.m. binge-watching cat videos instead of snoozing peacefully. That lack of sleep doesn't just leave you groggy—it also causes elevated cortisol levels, which leads to blood sugar spikes.

And it gets worse: Chronic sleep deprivation has been linked to increased appetite and cravings for sugary snacks—because who doesn't want a cookie at 3 a.m.? This insatiable desire for carbs can lead to overeating and weight gain, both of which are notorious contributors to type 2 diabetes. It's like trying to lose weight while standing in front of an all-you-can-eat buffet; the odds are not in your favor.

Studies show that individuals who go to bed after 11 p.m. may face more significant disruptions to their sleep quality and hormonal balance [Source 17]. Not only does this make it harder for your body to regulate blood sugar, but it also disrupts your body's natural hormonal rhythm. Hormones like melatonin, which help you fall asleep, peak in the hours leading up to midnight, so going to bed late can miss this window of optimal hormone release.

There's another factor that can make morning blood sugar levels tricky: the dawn phenomenon. If you've ever woken up with higher-than-usual blood sugar, even though you didn't eat anything overnight, you've probably experienced it. Between 3 a.m. and 8 a.m., your body releases a surge of hormones—like cortisol and growth hormone—to wake you up and get you moving. But this hormonal rush also signals your liver to dump glucose into the bloodstream, pushing blood sugar higher, even before breakfast [Source 18].

Patients used to ask me all the time, "Why is my blood sugar higher in the morning than when I went to bed, even though I didn't eat?" Well, it's like finishing the dishes before bed, only to find more magically appear in the sink while you're sleeping. So unfair, right? That's the dawn phenomenon at work—your body's way of releasing glucose into your bloodstream when you least expect it.

There's a simple fix: sleep timing is crucial for minimizing this. Going to bed earlier helps your body sync up its natural hormonal rhythms, reduce those morning glucose spikes, and keep blood sugar levels more stable throughout the day.

I can practically hear you now: "Okay, so when should I hit the sack to make this work? 10 p.m.? 10:30 p.m.? What's the magic number?" While everyone's sleep needs are different, the sweet spot is getting to bed before 11 p.m.—ideally between 9:30 and 10 p.m. Think of it as the prime time for your body to sync up with its natural circadian rhythm. This is when melatonin levels rise, deep sleep kicks in, and your body does its best restorative work. It also helps keep the release of growth hormone and cortisol on track, balancing everything from blood sugar to appetite. And here's a magic number you might be interested in: Research shows that getting at least seven hours of quality sleep each night can help stabilize blood glucose levels and reduce insulin resistance [Source 19]. The takeaway? Sleep isn't just for rest—it's your metabolic reset button.

But wait—there's more! It's not just about how long you sleep; it's about how well you sleep. Poor sleep quality isn't just an inconvenience—it's a serious metabolic issue. Studies show that bad sleep leads to higher blood glucose levels and worse control over blood sugar after meals (yes, that late-night snack might be doing more damage than you think) [Source 20]. In fact, research has found that people with fragmented sleep or insomnia have a significantly higher risk of developing type 2 diabetes compared to those who get a solid, uninterrupted night of rest [Source 21].

And here's where it gets even more interesting: deep sleep is a game-changer. It's the sleep stage that boosts insulin sensitivity. One study found that specific brain waves during deep sleep are actually tied to better blood sugar control the next day [Source 22]. So, if you're tossing and turning instead of hitting those deep sleep stages, you might be sabotaging your body's ability to manage glucose like a type zero diabetic.

So, what does all this mean for you? If you're serious about keeping your glucose levels in check and reducing your risk of prediabetes or diabetes, it's time to treat sleep like a priority—not a luxury. Just like a balanced diet and regular exercise, quality sleep should be non-negotiable. Aim for seven to nine hours of uninterrupted rest each night—trust me, your pancreas will thank you.

Start by embracing good sleep hygiene: establish a calming bedtime routine, ditch the screens (yes, even those cute cat videos), and transform your bedroom into a sleep sanctuary. Every hour of quality sleep is an investment in your metabolic health—think of it as giving your body a well-earned recharge.

In the end, while we may joke about our love-hate relationship with sleep (who hasn't hit snooze one too many times?), the truth is, the stakes are high. So let's raise our pillows (not our stress levels) and toast to sweet dreams, stable blood sugar, and a healthier future!

Stress: The Silent Sugar Saboteur

"Stress is like a rocking chair. It gives you something to do, but it doesn't get you anywhere."

— Anonymous

We've all been there—the tight deadlines, the never-ending emails, the constant juggling of kids' activities, or the stress of trying to keep that Instagram feed looking flawless (shoutout to all my Gen Z readers!). While we don't have saber-toothed tigers chasing us anymore, our modern-day stressors are pretty close: endless Zoom meetings, that unspoken pressure to reply to texts in under 30 seconds, and the quiet panic when you realize you've spent an hour scrolling through TikTok instead of actually relaxing.

And yet, when your boss pings you on Slack at 9 p.m. or you hear the constant buzz of notifications demanding your attention, your body's still reacting like it's running for its life. Stress hijacks your nervous system, and your brain signals your body to release a flood of hormones that scream *"fight or flight!"*

But instead of fleeing from a wild animal, we're running to the nearest coffee shop, grabbing that extra-large latte (because caffeine's totally going to solve everything, right?) and maybe a donut or two to keep us going (to give us a little "energy boost." And boom—there's that glucose spike.

Stress is a sneaky thing; it's not just about the big, obvious moments. It's those tiny, relentless stressors—the ones we barely notice—that add up to a full-blown blood sugar rollercoaster. Whether it's family drama or that constant buzz of notifications on your phone, stress does more than just make your heart race and your mind spin.

It triggers a hormonal storm, and the primary culprit is cortisol, the "stress hormone." When cortisol spikes, your body thinks it's in danger and needs to get ready for action. So, what does it do? It signals your liver to dump glucose into your bloodstream. This sudden influx of sugar is meant to give you the energy to fight or flee. However, we aren't designed to be in a constant state of high-alert stress. When we're in that "fight or flight" mode all the time, it takes a toll. Over time, those repeated blood sugar spikes can lead to insulin resistance and an increased risk of type 2 diabetes.

In fact, a landmark study revealed that individuals with high levels of work-related stress had a whopping 45% higher risk of developing type 2 diabetes compared to their less-stressed peers [Source 23]. Yep, stress isn't just an inconvenience—it's a serious player in your blood sugar game. And managing it? It's not optional. It's crucial for keeping your metabolism in check.

The Sleep-Stress-Sugar Triangle

Now, let's talk about the tricky triangle: sleep, stress, and blood sugar. It's like a three-way tug-of-war. Poor sleep spikes your stress, and high stress wrecks your sleep. Throw blood sugar into the mix, and boom—you've got a metabolic disaster on your hands. It's a vicious cycle, and I used to live and breathe this lifestyle—constantly stressed, never getting enough sleep, and wondering why my energy was all over the place.

Take, for example, a study by Chaput et al. (2013), which found that short sleep and bad sleep quality don't just cause exhaustion—they're linked to higher risks of obesity, type 2 diabetes, and even heart disease [Source 24]. And it doesn't stop there: stress makes everything worse. When you're stressed, your sleep quality takes a nosedive, your cortisol spikes, and your body becomes even more vulnerable to blood sugar problems. The bottom line is clear: when stress sabotages your sleep, the sleep-stress-sugar triangle goes into overdrive. That's when your blood sugar starts to spiral, and the damage piles up—insulin resistance, type 2 diabetes, weight gain... leading to a full-blown metabolic time bomb.

Breaking the Stress-Sugar Cycle: Practical Strategies for Balance

Now that we know the players, let's talk strategy. How do we break the cycle and get things back in balance? Here's what you can do to keep stress in check and your blood sugar stable:

Prioritize Sleep Hygiene: As you read above, aim for 7–9 hours of quality sleep every night. Research shows that just two weeks of better sleep—going from 7 to 14 days—can make a big difference in your blood sugar levels [Source 25]. It improves your body's ability to handle glucose and boosts insulin sensitivity, whether you have diabetes or not.

To make that happen, focus on creating a healthy pre-sleep routine— things like sticking to a regular sleep schedule (no sleeping until 11 a.m. on the weekends if you're waking up at 7 a.m. during the week), cutting out screens at least 30 minutes before bed (because scrolling through TikTok for "just five more minutes" never ends well), and creating a calm, cool sleep environment (now that I'm in menopause, I keep our bedroom at *Arctic-level* temperatures—my husband's basically buried under three blankets while I'm living my best polar bear life).

And if you think your afternoon caffeine habit isn't part of the equation, think again. Avoid caffeine after 2 p.m. (seriously, you won't even miss that second or third cup once you've got a solid sleep routine in place). Instead, try winding down with relaxing activities like reading (just maybe skip the thriller that'll have you glued to the pages at 1 a.m., trying to figure out who the killer is). Or, put on some calming music to set the mood before hitting the pillow. The more consistent you are with these habits, the better your chances of catching those restorative Zs.

Stress Management Techniques: The good news? You can actually lower those cortisol levels! Practices like meditation, mindfulness, and deep breathing are like the "Ctrl+Alt+Delete" for your stressed-out body. These simple techniques help calm your nervous system, reduce stress, and improve insulin sensitivity.

Instead of losing your mind over a deadline, take 10 minutes a day to just *breathe*—yes, I'm talking to you, an overachiever who's already thinking about the next 50 things you need to do (this used to be me!). Set a timer, close your eyes, and focus on your breath. It doesn't have to be a whole Zen experience—you don't need to be sitting cross-legged on a mountaintop in the Himalayas (unless that's your thing). Just 10 minutes of breathing and centering yourself can be a game-changer for your blood sugar.

And here's a bonus—when you manage stress, your brain gets a reset, too. You'll be more focused, less scatterbrained, and able to tackle that to-do list with expert efficiency.

Regular Physical Activity: Exercise is like the Swiss Army knife for your body—it's good for just about everything. It slashes stress, boosts insulin sensitivity, and keeps your blood sugar in check. Plus, it's a major mood booster. Whether you're taking a brisk walk (the kind where you're slightly breathless trying to talk to someone) or hitting the gym, it's a win for your body and mind.

Don't have time for a full workout? No problem. Research shows that even simple moves like squats or stretching at your desk can do wonders. A few squats during your lunch break—or when you're about to raid the pantry for candy, chips, or coffee in the afternoon—can lower cortisol and help your body handle blood sugar better. So, whether you've got 10 minutes or 30, your metabolism and mood will get the ultimate two-for-one: feel great and help your body work smarter.

When it comes to blood sugar management, diet and exercise get most of the glory. But don't overlook the behind-the-scenes heavy hitters: stress and sleep. Stress is the silent saboteur, and sleep? The unsung hero. By managing both, you're setting yourself up for metabolic success. When stress keeps popping up uninvited, take a breath, hit pause, and remember: Your body's metabolic balance is in your hands. And with a little attention to stress and sleep, you can turn your blood sugar's worst nightmare into a well-regulated dream. And if you're looking to level up your metabolism even further? Stick around— because in the next chapter, we're diving into how alternative diabetes defenders can give you that extra edge.

CHAPTER 6

Green Medicine: Herbal Hacks for Diabetes Prevention

"The best doctor gives the least medicine."

— Benjamin Franklin

W hen you hear the word "supplements," it's easy to picture a counter cluttered with endless bottles, each promising to solve everything from bloating to brain fog to blood sugar imbalances. I've lost count of the times patients have brought in bags full of pills—sometimes over 30 a day—and I've been left stunned. But here's the hard truth: not all supplements are created equal. Some are totally worth your time and money, while others? Well, they're just, as teens used to say, "extra."

Let's be clear: Herbs and natural supplements aren't the star of the show. They're your backup squad—stepping in after you've already put in the work with the strategies I cover in Chapters 3–5. Lifestyle medicine takes center stage, and green medicine works behind the scenes to give you that metabolic edge you need to truly thrive.

In this chapter, we're diving into my Top 10 List of supplements and herbs. These aren't the latest 2 a.m. infomercial gimmicks—they're the real deal, proven to support your health in meaningful ways. And because we're not into myths, I'll back up these claims with science, but in a way that doesn't require a PhD to understand.

Cinnamon: Not Just for Your Latte

Sure, cinnamon is delicious in your coffee or sprinkled on oatmeal, but it's also a powerhouse for blood sugar control. In fact, a 2013 study published in the *Journal of Medicinal Food* found that cinnamon helped improve insulin sensitivity, making it easier for your body to process glucose [Source 26]. The dose shown to help healthy adults respond better to insulin is 1 gram of cinnamon per day, which is about ½ teaspoon.

Keep in mind that the type of cinnamon matters—Ceylon cinnamon (also known as "true cinnamon") is preferred over cassia cinnamon, as it contains lower levels of coumarin, which could be harmful in large quantities.

Now, I'm not saying you should douse every meal in cinnamon (unless you want to walk around smelling like a cinnamon roll). But adding it to your smoothie, roasted vegetables, on apple slices, and in a chia seed pudding could provide some metabolic benefits. It's not a magic pill, but it certainly sweetens the deal when it comes to managing your blood sugar.

Turmeric: The Golden Wonder

You've probably heard that turmeric is great for inflammation, but did you know that it also has a profound impact on insulin resistance? A 2013 study in Diabetes Care revealed that curcumin, the active compound in turmeric, could reduce insulin resistance and help manage type 2 diabetes [Source 27].

Now, don't expect to get results by tossing turmeric on your morning eggs (unless you're into adventurous breakfasts). It's best absorbed when combined with black pepper (thanks to a compound called piperine), and ideally taken in supplement form or as part of a well-balanced recipe like a curry or smoothie.

If you choose to enjoy this in spice form, 1 to 3 teaspoons per day of turmeric powder is typically used in studies; in capsule form, 500 to 1,000 mg of curcumin per day is the common dose range in clinical studies aimed at improving insulin resistance.

You can also enjoy it as a turmeric latte or "golden milk" before bed [Source 28 for recipe]. This golden milk, used for centuries in Ayurvedic medicine, is not just a cozy treat but a wellness elixir that nurtures both body and mind. So, why not sip your way to better health?

Berberine: The Little Herb with Big Impact

If turmeric and cinnamon are the celebrities of the herbal world, then berberine is the quiet, unsung hero. It's been shown in several studies to help lower blood sugar and improve insulin sensitivity, sometimes even packing the same punch as metformin (the go-to diabetes drug).

A 2008 study in Metabolism found that berberine can significantly lower blood sugar levels in people with type 2 diabetes, proving it's definitely got some serious street cred in the supplement world [Source 29]. The magic dose? Around 500 mg to 1,500 mg per day, split up into 2 or 3 doses. Most studies suggest starting with 500 mg before meals to keep blood sugar in check after eating. Since it's best absorbed with food—especially carbs—take it with a meal for maximum impact.

A heads-up: Berberine can be a little rough on the stomach if you take too much at once, so it's best to divide the doses. Also, like turmeric, berberine has low bioavailability, so pairing it with piperine (from black pepper) can help it work its magic more effectively.

Magnesium: The Mineral We're All Missing

Alright, let's talk magnesium—the mineral that everyone says you're probably not getting enough of. Factors like chronic stress, poor diet, and certain medications (e.g., diuretics) can contribute to magnesium depletion. It's no wonder that 50–70% of people in the U.S. are running low on magnesium or living in that "suboptimal" zone.

Magnesium is famous for supporting muscle and nerve function, but it also plays a starring role in over 300 biochemical reactions in your body and is key when it comes to processing insulin. *The Journal of Clinical Endocrinology & Metabolism* found that magnesium deficiency is linked to a higher risk of type 2 diabetes [Source 30].

Clinical studies show that taking 250–500 mg per day of magnesium helps improve blood sugar control, especially if you're dealing with insulin resistance. Yes, you can eat more leafy greens and nuts, but honestly, it's a lot of work to get 250–500 mg of magnesium per day through food alone. You'd need to eat 3–4 servings of leafy greens, nuts, or seeds (plus a solid amount of whole grains) to hit that mark. If you're ambitious enough to work this into your daily diet, check out Source 31. For some of us, popping a supplement is a lot easier—and it works! If you're questioning which type of magnesium to get, pick magnesium citrate or glycinate—they're easier on your stomach and have better absorption.

Pro tip: Consider taking your magnesium at bedtime. Not only does it help you unwind and get a solid night's sleep, but it also gives your blood sugar and insulin levels a little nighttime TLC!

Alpha-Lipoic Acid (ALA): The Antioxidant for Your Cells

Alpha-Lipoic Acid (ALA) might not be a household name, but it's definitely a superstar when it comes to improving insulin sensitivity. Studies like the one published in The Journal of Clinical Investigation (2011) have shown that ALA can help reduce blood sugar levels and improve insulin function [Source 32].

But here's the catch: ALA isn't going to work its magic just by relying on food alone. To really see its magic in action, it's often best taken as a supplement. Clinical studies show that to get the full effect, you'd need to take 300 to 1,200 mg of ALA a day—and that's way more than what you'd find in your average spinach salad.

For example:

- To hit 300 mg of ALA, you'd need to eat several pounds of spinach or broccoli (definitely not the most appetizing meal plan).
- Organ meats (hello, liver) pack more ALA, but still, you'd have to eat several servings to match what's used in clinical studies.

Bottom line: While it's great to load up on ALA-rich foods (check out Source 33 for the full list), if you're really looking to boost your insulin sensitivity, a supplement is probably the way to go. It's a game-changer for your blood sugar, especially if you want to give your cells a little detox and put your metabolism on track.

Chromium: The Undercover Agent for Blood Sugar Control

Ah, chromium—the quiet superstar in the world of minerals. It doesn't get as much attention as its flashier cousins like magnesium and turmeric, but it sure knows how to pull its weight. Chromium plays a crucial role in glucose metabolism and is thought to help improve insulin sensitivity, making it a game-changer for blood sugar control.

Here's the science: A 2007 study published in *Diabetes Technology & Therapeutics* showed that chromium supplementation can boost insulin sensitivity in people with type 2 diabetes [Source 34]. Then, another study in the *Journal of Clinical Endocrinology & Metabolism* in 2016 confirmed that chromium helped lower blood sugar levels in people with insulin resistance [Source 35].

To hit those optimal blood sugar benefits, clinical studies typically recommend 200 mcg to 1,000 mcg (that's 1 mg) of chromium per day. Sounds simple, right? Well, not so fast.

Sure, you can find it in foods like broccoli, whole grains, and meats (for the full list, check out Source 36), but to get the minimum 200 mcg, you'd have to eat 9 cups of cooked broccoli, 20 slices of whole wheat bread, and 67–100 ounces of meat, respectively—and let's be honest, that's a bit much to pack into a day!

So, as with ALA, while incorporating chromium-rich foods can be part of a healthy diet, taking a chromium supplement could be your ticket to better blood sugar management and the secret weapon your routine has been missing.

Apple Cider Vinegar: Not Just for Salad Anymore

When you think of apple cider vinegar, your mind might immediately go to those TikTok videos of people swishing it around in their mouths (don't do that, by the way) or the faint memory of Grandma swearing by it for everything from digestion to detox. But the truth is, there's real scientific data behind its blood sugar benefits—so it's not just all hype.

Let's break it down: A 2004 study published in Diabetes Care found that vinegar improved insulin sensitivity in subjects with insulin resistance or type 2 diabetes [Source 37]. Another recent study published in Frontiers in Nutrition found that taking ACV (apple cider vinegar) daily can actually *lower fasting blood sugar* and improve insulin sensitivity—two big wins for reducing your risk of type 2 diabetes [Source 38].

In fact, people who took at least 3 teaspoons of apple cider vinegar daily for two months saw their fasting blood sugar drop by about **22 points**, and their A1c (a long-term blood sugar marker) dropped by up to **1.5%**—which is a big deal in diabetes prevention.

How does it work? It's believed that acetic acid, the active compound in apple cider vinegar, may help block the digestion of starches, thereby slowing down the absorption of sugar into the bloodstream.

This means you're less likely to get those sharp, high spikes in blood sugar after a meal.

But wait, it gets better. A 2024 study published in *BMJ Nutrition, Prevention & Health* found that daily consumption of apple cider vinegar led to significant reductions in weight, body mass index, waist/hip circumferences, and body fat ratio in individuals with overweight and obesity [Source 39]. So, you get the double whammy of helping your blood sugar and supporting your metabolism.

Now, before you go chugging shots of ACV like it's your new energy drink (please don't), there's a better way to incorporate it into your routine. Aim for about 1–2 tablespoons diluted in water, preferably before meals, or use it as a base for your salad dressing. And, of course, if you're on medication, talk to your healthcare provider first, as apple cider vinegar can have interactions with certain diabetic drugs (causing hypoglycemia), diuretics (causing low potassium), and ACE inhibitors (causing high potassium).

Vitamin D: Sunshine in a Capsule (For Your Blood Sugar, Too)

We all know vitamin D is a key player in keeping our bones strong, but here's a fun fact: it also helps with blood sugar regulation! A study published in the *Journal of Clinical Endocrinology & Metabolism* found that vitamin D deficiency is closely linked to insulin resistance and higher blood sugar levels [Source 40]. In fact, if your vitamin D levels are low, you're at a higher risk for developing type 2 diabetes.

So, how do you keep your levels in check? To optimize glucose metabolism and insulin sensitivity, aim for a vitamin D level between

50 ng/mL and 70 ng/mL on your blood tests. This sweet spot has been linked to better insulin sensitivity, a lower risk of type 2 diabetes, and overall health benefits.

The effective dose of vitamin D depends on factors like your age, baseline levels, and health conditions. While 1,000 to 2,000 IU per day is typical, some people may need more to hit that optimal level. The best way to know for sure? Get the 25-hydroxyvitamin D test to check your current levels.

Now, about the sunshine factor: the amount of sun exposure you need to keep those levels up depends on things like your skin tone, where you live, and the time of year. Here's a general guide:

- 10 to 30 minutes of sun exposure on bare skin (like your arms, legs, or face) a few times a week is usually enough.
- Fair-skinned folks might need less (10–15 minutes), while those with darker skin may need 30 minutes to an hour or more.
- Best time to soak up the rays? Between 10 a.m. and 4 p.m., when UVB rays are strongest.

Things to keep in mind:

- Latitude & Season: If you're far from the equator or living in a colder climate, you may need supplements in winter when the sun peeks out rarely.
- Sunscreen: While it's a must for protecting your skin, it can block vitamin D production. Try short bursts of sun exposure (about 10–15 minutes) without it—just don't forget to reapply later!

Pro tip: As you age, your ability to make vitamin D from sunlight might dip, and more clothes mean less skin exposure, so be sure to keep an eye on your levels and consider supplementation if needed.

If you're not getting enough rays, a good vitamin D supplement can help boost your insulin sensitivity and give your metabolism a little sunshine, without the risk of a sunburn!

Zinc: More Than Just a Cold Remedy

Zinc isn't just your go-to for fighting off colds—it's a total game-changer when it comes to managing blood sugar! Research from the *International Journal of Vitamin and Nutrition Research* has shown that zinc plays a crucial role in insulin function and glucose metabolism [Source 41]. In fact, people with diabetes often have lower zinc levels, and studies have found that supplementing with zinc can help improve insulin sensitivity.

For optimal blood sugar control, the recommended dose is typically between **20 and 40 mg** per day. And here's a fun fact: Oysters are the ultimate zinc powerhouse—just a few ounces will give you a big zinc boost. But don't worry, there are other zinc-rich foods, like beef, pumpkin seeds, and chickpeas (you can find the full list in Source 42).

Now, while it's tough to hit that sweet spot through food alone, zinc supplements might be a smart move if you're focused on improving blood sugar or insulin resistance. Just keep in mind, too much zinc can lead to side effects like nausea and interfere with copper absorption. So, as always, be sure to chat with your healthcare provider before jumping on the zinc bandwagon. Your body will thank you for the extra support—just make sure you're doing it the right way!

Omega-3s: Fat That Loves Your Metabolism

Omega-3 fatty acids aren't just a treat for your heart—they're also a powerful ally in managing diabetes! Studies, like one published in *Diabetes Care*, show that omega-3s can reduce insulin resistance, meaning your body can use insulin more efficiently [Source 43]. How? By tackling inflammation, which is a major culprit behind insulin resistance.

So, how much do you need? Aiming for 1,000 to 2,000 milligrams (1–2 grams) of omega-3s a day is the sweet spot for supporting blood sugar balance and insulin sensitivity. And you know why everyone's slapping chia and hemp seeds on everything? Because they're packed with omega-3s! Check out Source 44 for a full list of omega-3-rich foods and how much to eat.

Just when you thought that was it: Omega-3s are champs at lowering triglycerides. Why does that matter? Because high triglycerides don't just mess with your heart, they also crank up your risk for diabetes. When you use omega-3s to keep your triglycerides in check, you're hitting two major health goals at once—it's a win for your heart and a win for your blood sugar.

If you're not a fan of fish or flaxseeds, omega-3 supplements like fish oil are an easy go-to. Typically, 1–2 soft gels can give you the necessary dose. Just remember, it can be tough to hit your omega-3 goals with food alone, especially if you're not eating fatty fish regularly. So, if you're looking to "hook" that perfect blood sugar balance, a supplement might just be the catch of the day!

The Bottom Line: Supplements as Your Secret Weapon

There you have it—botanical boosts that are more than just Instagram-worthy. Herbs and supplements may seem like the shortcut to better health, but here's the deal: they work best when paired with a solid diet and exercise routine. They're not magic pills, but they serve as powerful sidekicks in your health journey. Think of them like your wingmen, always there to support your body in ways food and exercise alone might miss. But here's the catch: consistency is everything. You won't see results by just sprinkling a little cinnamon on your oats one day or taking a magnesium pill on a random Wednesday. These herbs and supplements need to become part of your daily routine to really make an impact.

Next time you're eyeing the supplement aisle or getting swept up in the latest wellness craze, remember: not every new bottle is a shortcut to health nirvana. But with the right herbs and supplements on your team, you can level up your blood sugar and metabolism game. Now, you've got the goods—diet, exercise, sleep, stress management, and supplements. Next, we'll turn that powerhouse combo into your secret weapon and crush those glucose and insulin levels like a boss. It's go time!

CHAPTER 7

Mission Possible: Your Diabetes-Defeating Battle Plan

"If you know the enemy and know yourself, you need not fear the results of a hundred battles."

— Sun Tzu

Alright, sugar warrior, it's time to put those theories into action and turn you into a diabetes-fighting machine. Think of this chapter as your ultimate game plan—the grocery list, meal prep strategy, and survival tactics that'll have you slaying prediabetes (or diabetes) without breaking a sweat. No more excuses, no more sugar crashes. Just pure, unfiltered victory. And the first weapon you'll want to load up on? Fiber—your secret weapon in the battle for steady blood sugar.

Fiber: The Mighty Weapon You've Been Overlooking

The average American is getting only about 15 grams of fiber a day, well below the recommended 30 to 40 grams. Why? It's no mystery. Our busy, fast-paced lives lead us to grab whatever's convenient, often opting for processed snacks and quick meals that are low in fiber. For example, a bowl of Raisin Bran cereal (which *sounds* healthy because of the "bran," until you discover the 20 grams of sugar in those raisins). Or maybe it's a Starbucks pastry or a Dunkin' Donut, which will give you a quick sugar rush followed by a crash that leaves you craving more junk. And that McDonald's value meal—sure, it's a "deal," but it's *not* valuing your health. Or chips, those crispy, salty little nuggets of empty calories that leave you feeling satisfied for about 30 seconds before you reach for another handful. These quick-fix foods may seem convenient, but they often skimp on fiber while packing in processed carbs and sugar. And that fiber deficit? It's quietly wreaking havoc on our blood sugar, metabolism, and overall health.

Now, for those over 50, fiber recommendations get a little more nuanced. As we age, digestion can slow down (hello, bloating and gas), staying hydrated becomes trickier (fiber needs plenty of water to do its job), and conditions like diverticulitis can make too much fiber a no-go. It's all about striking that perfect balance! Now that you're armed with the fiber facts, it's time to take action! Let's dive into the first weapon on our Battle Plan Grocery List—veggies!

The Type Zero Diabetic Grocery List

Veggies: The Good, The Better, and the Glucose-Busting Best!

You'd think shopping for vegetables would be a no-brainer, right? But here's the sneaky thing: some veggies "appear" healthy, but when you take a closer look, they have a surprisingly high amount of carbs and sugar. The trick is to focus on the veggies with the best macro balance: low in carbs, low in sugar, but packing a serious fiber punch. Ready for your top 10 veggie lineup? Here you go:

- Spinach – Fiber: 4g, Net Carbs: 1g, Sugar: 0.4g
  It's the MVP of fiber and low in carbs and sugar. Bulk up your meals without raising your blood sugar.
- Broccoli – Fiber: 5g, Net Carbs: 4g, Sugar: 1.5g
  This all-star veggie is not just for looks; it's loaded with fiber and antioxidants.
- Cauliflower – Fiber: 3g, Net Carbs: 2g, Sugar: 1.9g
  Need a rice or potato substitute? Cauliflower's got your back, keeping it low on carbs and sugar.
- Zucchini – Fiber: 2g, Net Carbs: 2g, Sugar: 3.5g
  Zucchini's like the chameleon of veggies. Low-carb noodles, stir-fries, or just as a snack—take your pick.
- Asparagus – Fiber: 3g, Net Carbs: 3g, Sugar: 2.5g
  Packed with fiber and minimal sugar, asparagus is a low-carb sidekick to your protein.
- Brussels Sprouts – Fiber: 4g, Net Carbs: 5g, Sugar: 2g
  Bite-sized, fiber-packed, and nutrient-rich—this veggie is just bursting with goodness.
- Green Beans – Fiber: 4g, Net Carbs: 4g, Sugar: 2.4g
  These little beans pack a punch in fiber while keeping net carbs nice and low. Toss them in salads or as a side dish.
- Cabbage – Fiber: 5g, Net Carbs: 3g, Sugar: 3.2g
  Cabbage is the versatile veggie that shows up in everything from slaws to stir-fries. And it won't spike your blood sugar.
- Kale – Fiber: 3g, Net Carbs: 3g, Sugar: 0.5g
  Another leafy green to love—high in fiber, low in carbs, and oh-so-tasty in smoothies or soups.

- Mushrooms – Fiber: 1g, Net Carbs: 2g, Sugar: 1g

  Mushrooms are low in carbs, low in sugar, and add that meaty texture we all crave. They're the quiet fiber powerhouse of your plate.

Now, let's talk about those veggies that sneak in more carbs and sugar than we'd like, while skimping on fiber. Yep, we're talking potatoes (both white and sweet—sadly, sweet potatoes aren't the miracle low-carb veggie we hoped for), corn, carrots, beets, peas, and butternut squash. The key here? Portion control. For example, I'll nibble on 6–7 baby carrots or toss half a small sweet potato into a breakfast hash with eggs and spinach. Also, try to enjoy these veggie carb bombs earlier in the day—breakfast or lunch, not dinner. Why? Because when you eat high-carb veggies earlier, your metabolism has time to burn those carbs before the evening slows you down. After dinner, let's face it, most of us aren't taking a brisk walk, and those sugars will stick around longer, possibly messing with your blood sugar balance while you sleep. Keep the portions small and keep it early!

Fats that Fuel: Supercharge Your Sugar Control

Let's talk about healthy fats—your blood sugar's best friend when it comes to staying steady and supporting insulin sensitivity. These fats slow down sugar absorption into your bloodstream, keeping those blood sugar spikes and crashes at bay, and helping you avoid that hangry feeling.

Healthy fats come from delicious sources like avocados, nuts, seeds, olive oil, and fatty fish like salmon. They help regulate the absorption of carbs and keep your energy steady throughout the day. But don't go overboard—no olive oil baths here! Instead, think of small but powerful additions: a handful of almonds (12–15 pieces) for a snack, a drizzle of olive oil on your salad, 2–3 slices of avocado on your toast, or a 5-ounce portion of salmon with your meal. Easy, right?

Now, if you're wondering how much fat your body actually needs, clinical studies suggest 25% to 35% of your daily calories should come from fat to help prevent diabetes and heart disease. However, let's get real—not all fats are created equal. You'll want to limit saturated fats to under 10% of your total calories. So, if you're chowing down on bacon, butter, or cheese, it's time to pump the brakes. And trans fats? Just. Say. No. These artificial fats hide out in packaged snacks, fried foods, and baked goods—best to skip them completely.

The bottom line: Healthy fats don't just love your heart; they help keep your blood sugar in check, too. Keep the good fats, ditch the bad ones, and your heart, insulin levels, and energy will thank you!

Building a Diabetes-Free Future with Whole Grains

Whole grains are total rock stars when it comes to keeping your blood sugar on track and keeping prediabetes or diabetes at bay. And guess what? Adding them to your daily routine is way easier than you think. Start small—swap that plain bagel and cream cheese for a slice of Dave's Killer Bread topped with avocado and an egg. Instant upgrade! You'll get fiber, healthy fats, and protein, without the blood sugar spike.

Whole grains like oats, quinoa, brown rice, and barley give you steady energy and keep you full longer, without that post-carb crash. But here's the key: don't eat them solo. Pair your grains with protein and veggies to really stabilize your blood sugar. Try a quinoa bowl with grilled chicken and roasted veggies, or mix oats with chia seeds and almond butter for a killer breakfast. Also, eating your whole grains earlier in the day works wonders since your metabolism is more active.

Now, let's take a quick peek at what to swap out in your pantry. These easy exchanges can help you boost your intake of whole grains, fiber, and protein while still enjoying similar tastes and textures to the foods you're used to!

1. White Potatoes → Sweet Potatoes, Butternut Squash, or even Cauliflower (mashed or "rice," it's delicious!)
2. White Bread → Whole Wheat or Sprouted Grain Bread
3. White Rice → Brown Rice, Wild Rice, or Quinoa (protein-packed and fiber-rich)
4. Regular Pasta → High-Protein Pasta (made from lentils, chickpeas, or edamame) or Zoodles (because zucchini makes everything better)
5. Sugary Cereals → High-Fiber Cereal (think bran flakes, shredded wheat, or oats)
6. Regular Pancakes → Whole Wheat or Protein Pancakes (bonus points for adding Greek yogurt)

Now let's put this practice—here are my Top 10 real-life, simple swaps you can start making today that'll have a big impact on keeping your blood sugar in check and supporting your health.

1. Regular oatmeal → High-protein, low-carb oatmeal (no more than ½ cup and add cinnamon instead of brown sugar for flavor)
2. Honey Nut Cheerios → Plain Cheerios with ¼ cup fresh blueberries (more fiber, less sugar)

3. White rice → ½ cup brown rice or quinoa (higher fiber, more nutrients) at lunch, not dinner

4. Regular pasta → ½ cup high-protein pasta made with lentils, chickpeas, or edamame at lunch, not dinner (more protein, fewer carbs)

5. Russet baked potato → half of a small sweet potato with cinnamon and nutmeg (no brown sugar, just natural sweetness)

6. White bread → 1 slice (you don't need 2 slices!) whole-grain, high-fiber bread (Dave's Killer Bread is a great option!)

7. Bagel with cream cheese → half of a whole wheat English muffin (you don't need the whole English muffin!) with 2 tbsp peanut butter (healthy fats and protein)

8. Regular granola → ¼ cup low-sugar granola or make your own with nuts, seeds, and a sprinkle of cinnamon (but keep it less than ⅓ cup)

9. Regular crackers → Whole grain crackers (my favorite are Wasa—higher fiber, more filling, so you only need 1–2)

10. Store-bought granola bars → High protein, high fiber protein bars (I enjoy occasionally a Quest or Pure Protein bar, half of a bar as a snack, and the entire bar as a meal replacement)

I hope you can see now that you don't need to fear or ditch carbs altogether. I have been enjoying carbs while continuing to enjoy living the Type Zero Diabetic life and have never felt deprived. You now have the tools to build a diabetes-free future by choosing smarter whole grain options and being mindful of portions, timing, and pairings. When these simple swaps and mindset shifts become part of your new lifestyle, you'll keep your blood sugar in check, feel energized, and still enjoy all your favorite foods. It's all about balance—and you're in control!

Power Up with Protein: The Smarter Way to Master Your Blood Sugars

Protein is your ultimate sidekick in the fight against blood sugar chaos. Not only does it help keep blood sugar levels stable, but it also keeps you feeling full longer—goodbye, carb cravings! Whether it's lean chicken, turkey, tofu, or beans, adding more protein to your meals builds muscle, burns fat, and supports metabolic health. It's like hitting a triple whammy—muscle gain, fat loss, and better glucose control. And here's the best part—protein also boosts insulin sensitivity, keeps inflammation low, and even releases GLP-1, the same hormone found in expensive diabetes medications like Ozempic (but without the price tag, the weekly injections, and the side effects!). So load up on lean proteins, take charge of your health, and let your body do the heavy lifting. It's a win-win for your muscles and your metabolism!

Making smarter protein choices is easier than you think. Here are 10 simple swaps to go from fatty to lean and mean:

- Skinless Chicken Breast instead of Fried Chicken
- Turkey Bacon instead of Pork Bacon
- Lean Ground Turkey (93% lean or higher) instead of Regular Ground Beef
- Grilled or Baked Fish instead of Fried Fish
- Chicken Sausage instead of Pork Sausage
- Baked or Grilled Chicken Thighs instead of Fried Chicken Thighs
- Tuna in Water instead of Tuna in Oil
- Lean Beef (like Sirloin) instead of Ribeye
- Sauteed Shrimp instead of Fried Shrimp
- Tempeh or Tofu instead of Bacon

Here are the top lean proteins you definitely want on your grocery list—and why each one is a powerhouse for building muscle, boosting insulin sensitivity, stabilizing blood sugar, fighting inflammation, and trimming that excess fat:

Skinless Chicken Breast

- Benefits: Helps stabilize blood sugar, improves insulin sensitivity, and supports lean muscle mass development.

Turkey Breast

- Benefits: Supports muscle mass, improves metabolic function, and provides essential nutrients like B vitamins that aid in glucose metabolism.

Fish (Salmon, Cod, Tuna, and Sardines)

- Benefits: Reduces inflammation, improves insulin sensitivity, and supports cardiovascular health. Fatty fish like salmon can help with fat loss and improve muscle mass due to the healthy fats.

Lean Beef (Sirloin, Tenderloin)

- Benefits: Helps build muscle mass, supports healthy metabolism, and contains nutrients that help with insulin regulation.

Egg Whites

- Benefits: Supports muscle recovery and growth, helps stabilize blood sugar levels, and is great for those looking to control fat intake while maintaining muscle mass.

Greek Yogurt (Non-fat or Low-fat)

- Benefits: Reduces inflammation, supports muscle health, stabilizes blood sugar, and helps regulate appetite.

Tofu

- Benefits: Supports muscle growth, reduces inflammation, and helps stabilize blood sugar. It also contains phytoestrogens that may support metabolic health.

Tempeh

- Benefits: High in fiber and protein, tempeh can help with weight management, improve insulin sensitivity, and reduce inflammation. It's a great alternative for muscle maintenance in plant-based diets.

Cottage Cheese (Low-fat or Fat-free)

- Benefits: Helps with muscle repair and growth, supports fat loss due to its low-calorie content, and aids in insulin sensitivity.

Lentils and Beans

- Benefits: Help regulate blood sugar levels, reduce inflammation, and improve insulin sensitivity. They are also a great option for muscle building when combined with other protein sources.

Bison

- Benefits: Supports muscle mass, helps with fat loss, and provides important nutrients like iron and zinc to support overall metabolic health.

Lean Pork (Tenderloin or Loin Chop)

- Benefits: Provides a rich source of protein and essential nutrients, supports muscle building, and helps regulate blood sugar levels.

Now you're probably wondering, "Okay, but how much protein should I be eating a day?" Here's the deal: the amount of protein you need to stabilize glucose and improve insulin sensitivity depends on:

- Body weight and muscle mass (the more you weigh and the more muscle you have, the more protein you may need to help maintain or build muscle, and the better your body will be at using glucose efficiently)
- Activity level (exercise, especially resistance or strength training, increases your protein needs since it helps build muscle and improves insulin sensitivity)
- Age (as we age, our bodies become less efficient at utilizing protein, so we need more to maintain muscle mass and prevent sarcopenia/muscle loss)
- Health conditions (like prediabetes, obesity, or hormonal issues like thyroid issues or PCOS)
- Your specific goals (muscle building or fat loss)
- Timing and distribution of meals (eating protein at every meal can prevent glucose spikes and improve insulin sensitivity, and having protein post-workout helps with muscle repair/recovery and insulin sensitivity)
- Carb intake and overall diet quality (when you're on a low-carb diet, you need to compensate with slightly higher protein intake to make sure you're getting enough energy and supporting muscle growth and repair)

- Protein source and quality (lean proteins, like the ones listed above, are better at supporting muscle and managing glucose than fatty or processed meats)
- Lifestyle factors like stress, sleep, and gut health (did you know a healthy gut can help you absorb nutrients from protein more efficiently, which can aid in stabilizing blood sugar?)

I know that's A LOT of factors to consider when you're trying to figure out how much protein you should have! If you would like a personalized amount calculated just for you, schedule a complimentary Strategy Call on my website drhormonehacker.com to find out. In the meantime, here is a quick breakdown to guide you:

- For better insulin sensitivity: A little extra protein can go a long way. Aim for 1.2 to 1.5 grams per kilogram (or 0.54 to 0.68 grams per pound). For a 150-pound person, that's roughly 80 to 100 grams per day.
- For muscle and weight management: If you're lifting weights or shedding fat, you might need more. Studies suggest 1.6 to 2.2 grams per kilogram (about 0.73 to 1 gram per pound) will support muscle growth and help manage glucose. For a 150-pound person, that's about 110 to 135 grams per day.

A good place to start is 1.0 to 1.2 grams per kilogram if you're focused on stabilizing glucose and improving insulin sensitivity. Then, increase it gradually from there based on your health needs. And remember, spreading your protein intake throughout the day—especially if you're working out—gives you the best bang for your buck. You've got this!

With the right protein on your plate, you're not just controlling your blood sugar—you're owning your health and mastering the Type Zero Diabetic lifestyle. Now, let's get smart about meal prep so you're always ready to stay on track, whether you're slammed at work or living it up on vacation.

Meal and Mindset Prep: Outsmarting Your Future Hungry Self

Here's the deal: future-you is sneaky. When you're running on low energy or dealing with a busy schedule, that pick-me-up sugary coffee and pastry or afternoon chips and dip or pizza for dinner starts looking very inviting. So, let's beat future-you to the punch with some solid meal prep.

Sunday (Or Whatever Day You Choose) Prep Party

Pick a day—any day—and become your own meal prep pro. Chop those veggies, cook protein in bulk, and portion out your whole grains like brown rice or quinoa. Keep it simple with healthy dishes like salads, grain bowls, or roasted veggies, and have them ready to go for the week. Personally, I boil 8–10 eggs and bake a few chicken breasts, or I'll shred a rotisserie chicken for easy meals throughout the week. Don't want to roast veggies? No problem. I sauté spinach in two minutes, or I microwave frozen veggies. The easiest solution is to open a pre-packed salad (just be mindful of the dressing and skip the sugary dried fruit) and dump a can of tuna on top (I've done this many nights and it's quick and delish!). Trust me, you'll thank yourself at 6 p.m. when you're starving, and your only options are an unhealthy drive-thru or a quick bowl of cereal—both of which will have you riding a sugar high and crash in an hour.

The Smart Snack Stash

Having healthy snacks on hand is like having a secret stash of ammo for when hunger strikes. I keep individual servings of nuts (10–12 raw almonds are my go-to), string cheese, a tangerine, those cute hummus packs with baby carrots, or Greek yogurt cups (Triple Zero Oikos or low-sugar Chobani are my staples). Keeping these in your pantry, fridge, or even in your car will save you from the temptation of a handful of cheese and crackers (yep, I've been there), a candy bar, or a pit stop for small fries and a diet soda.

The "Leftovers Are Life" Strategy

I grew up fighting my brothers for the last bit of leftovers my mom made, especially since her cooking always tasted even better the next day. Leftovers aren't just for lazy days—they're a total game-changer. Repurpose last night's dinner into a killer lunch or turn that grilled chicken into a quick salad with fresh veggies and vinaigrette, wrap it in a tortilla with cheese and salsa, or even make a chicken salad sandwich. Got extra roasted veggies? Blend them into a soup with broth, toss them in an egg scramble, or mix them with pasta and pesto for a quick side dish. Leftover cooked rice? Stir-fry it with veggies and protein for a fried rice meal or use it in a rice bowl with different toppings. Leftover quinoa? Perfect for a grain bowl with fresh veggies and that extra piece of salmon you had the other night. Eating healthy doesn't have to take forever, and leftovers are your secret weapon.

Feast Smart, Celebrate Big

Ah, the holiday season. It's a parade of pies, cookies, and that legendary stuffing everyone raves about. Or maybe you're headed to your friend's house for an authentic Italian or Asian feast—delicious, but heavy on the carbs. Not exactly blood sugar-friendly, right? Don't worry! You can still indulge and enjoy the festivities without the sugar spike. Here's how to navigate these tasty landmines with ease.

No need to completely skip out on the good stuff and feel deprived, but if you're heading to a party, set yourself up for success by planning ahead! Ask what's on the menu and offer to bring a healthy dish—vegetable sides always hit the mark. If you're flying blind, have some protein and veggies before you go so you're not starving when you arrive, diving straight into the chips and spinach artichoke dip.

Here are a few easy swaps to help keep your blood sugar in check: opt for sweet potatoes instead of mashed potatoes (more fiber, fewer carbs), salsa over creamy dips (fresh, low-carb, and a little zesty), mixed nuts instead of Chex mix (fewer carbs, same crunch), and pumpkin pie instead of pecan pie (less sugar, still delicious). Make smart choices and keep those portions in check, and yep—you can totally have your cake and eat it, too (2–3 bites, that is)!

Speaking of smart portions, here are some simple visuals to keep in mind:

- 1 cup = your fist
- ½ cup = half a baseball
- ¼ cup = 1 golf ball
- 3 oz = the size of a deck of cards
- 1 tablespoon = 1 thumb

By making a few smart choices, you can enjoy the holiday or attend dinner parties without sacrificing your health goals.

Navigating Menus Like a Blood Sugar Pro

If you're heading out to eat, take a peek at the menu before you go and choose options that align with your goals. Trust me, my husband knows I've already picked out my salad and entrée before we even walk in. And whatever you do, don't skip breakfast to "save room" for a big meal—it always backfires. Start your day with something light and balanced, like egg and avocado toast, to keep your energy steady.

If you're facing a buffet of doom, choose your priorities. Fill up on veggies and protein first, so they're each 40% of your plate, then add carbs to the remaining 20% of your plate. Then, after waiting at least 15 minutes (the time it takes your brain to get the signal from your stomach that you're full) and having a tall glass of water, only if you're still hungry, go for a small portion of your favorite indulgence.

The Art of Drinking: Stay Hydrated, Time It Right, and Keep Your Blood Sugar in Check

Alcohol can definitely be a tricky one when it comes to managing blood sugar. Those sugary cocktails like margarita, cosmopolitan, and sangria? Total sugar bombs in disguise—they'll spike your blood sugar faster than you can say "cheers." Instead, if you choose to have alcohol, go for lighter options like wine, a vodka soda, or a gin and tonic. If you're borderline prediabetic or diabetic, consider going dry for a while or cutting back on alcohol to really notice the difference.

And here's the game-changer: keep water in the mix. Drinking water between alcoholic beverages can help keep blood sugar levels in check by:

1. slowing down alcohol absorption

2. preventing dehydration, which can increase the concentration of glucose in the blood

3. reducing the risk of alcohol overconsumption by helping you feel fuller and more satisfied

A well-hydrated, clear-headed you is unstoppable—and sometimes taking a break from alcohol altogether is the best way to stay focused on your health goals.

Here's another potential game-changer: timing your alcohol. To help optimize glucose and insulin metabolism, aim to stop drinking at least 2–3 hours before bed (but don't get the idea you can stay up until 3 a.m. just because you stopped at midnight—more on that in Chapter 5). Giving your body this extra time to process alcohol helps prevent nighttime blood sugar dips (hypoglycemia!) and supports better sleep. Plus, drinking earlier in the evening sets you up for more stable blood sugar levels overnight and can reduce those hangover nasties like dehydration, fatigue, and headaches the next day. A few small shifts in when and how much you drink can have a big impact on your blood sugar control!

Vacation Mode: How to Have a Sweet Getaway

Vacation mode: ON! It's all about relaxing, not stressing over every meal. But here's the thing: You can still enjoy your time away without letting your blood sugar take a vacation, too. Go for fresh seafood, grilled chicken, or a vibrant salad instead of that heavy pasta or fried dish. Want dessert? Go for it—but keep it in check with just 2–3 bites and share it with family and friends (remember that you get the most pleasure from the first 2–3 bites). Keep water with you at all times— whether you're lounging in the sun, hiking, or sightseeing. Make sure you're getting protein at every meal to avoid reaching for chips and salsa or snacking on your kids' chicken fingers by the pool (guilty!). Stay active by opting for the stairs instead of the elevator, or enjoy a leisurely walk around the hotel after dinner. The vacation vibe is all about balance, not guilt. Focus on creating memories with the people you love, make smart choices when you can, and indulge in the things you truly crave (not just what's in front of you). When you get home, jump right back into your groove and keep crushing it!

Here's the real secret sauce: Consistency is your superpower. Armed with your grocery list, meal prep hacks, and a solid game plan, you're ready to own this journey—no matter what life or the holidays throw your way. You've got the tools, the knowledge, and the strategy to make smarter choices. But here's the key: Don't try to change everything all at once. That's a fast track to overwhelm and burnout. Focus on 1–2 small action steps, nail them, and then move on to the next. Don't let hesitation hold you back—the sooner you get your plan into motion, the sooner you'll start seeing the results that stack the odds in your favor. So, kick things off right now—one healthy meal, workout, and stress-free moment at a time.

Now that you're in the driver's seat, let's dive into how you can rewrite the rules and break the chains of diabetes—because this battle? You're about to redefine the game.

CHAPTER 8

Rewrite the Rules: How Type Zero Breaks the Chains of Diabetes

"Learn the rules of the game; then play better than everyone else." — Albert Einstein

Think about how Las Vegas casinos always seem to win, no matter how lucky the gambler feels. The house has studied every little detail: how many drinks to serve to loosen up their players, when to increase the stakes, and even what time of night people are most likely to make risky bets. They know the habits, the vulnerabilities, and the sweet spots that keep gamblers coming back to lose again and again. The odds are always stacked in their favor.

Now, picture diabetes as the house. It's been studying your body just like a casino studies its gamblers. It knows how your body reacts to that plate of pasta, the slice of bread, the mashed potatoes, and those late-night sweets. Diabetes tracks how inactive and sedentary you are after sitting at a desk all day, how your energy drops when you're running on fumes after a 1 a.m. Netflix binge, and how your body struggles to process everything it's being fed. Slowly but surely, diabetes starts to craft its own winning strategy.

But here's the game-changer: you can still win. You may not be able to beat Vegas, but with early detection and smart, preventative lifestyle changes, you can hit the jackpot with your future health. By making small, intentional changes now—whether it's adjusting your diet, staying active, or getting quality sleep—you're taking control of the game. Diabetes won't know what hit it.

It's time to flip the script on diabetes. You've been fed the narrative that this is a battle you can't win. Well, it's time to burn that playbook and write your own rules. Type Zero is not just a lifestyle; it's a mindset that shatters the old patterns and sets you on a path to total control. You're not just managing your health; you're owning it.

This isn't about settling for "good enough" or "it could be worse." It's about rewriting the game entirely. You've got the tools to take charge and make diabetes play by your rules. And here's the kicker: when you break free from the chains of diabetes, you're not just improving your blood sugar—you're transforming every aspect of your health: from sharper focus to higher energy, to reducing your risk of complications like heart disease, kidney failure, and nerve damage.

But here's where it gets even bigger: when you take control of your health, you're not just breaking the chains for yourself. You're doing it for your kids, your siblings, your cousins, aunts, uncles, parents, and grandparents. The people you care about. Your new choices and lifestyle can spark a revolutionary ripple effect—one that shifts the entire trajectory of your family's health for generations. I missed my chance to live the Type Zero lifestyle in time to guide my grandmother, aunt, and mother—to help them improve their health, and maybe even prevent or reverse their diabetes.

That chance is gone—and I'll carry that forever.

But *you* still can.

Don't wait. Don't stay silent.

Be the messenger. Be the hope. Be the spark. Be the example.

Your loved ones are watching—and you might be their only shot at real change.

When it comes to exercise, I always ask my patients and clients two straightforward questions about the gym: 1) Do you belong to a gym? 2) How often do you actually go? If they tell me they're "members" but haven't set foot in the gym for months, I don't mince words: "You're not a member, you're a donor."

Let me make something crystal clear: there are no donors in the Type Zero Diabetic Club. Your membership isn't handed to you—it's earned with every choice you make, every meal you plan, and every drop of sweat you put in. It's earned with every piece of fresh, healthy food you pile on your plate, no matter what your friends or family are munching on. It's earned with every day you push through the exhaustion and move your body, even when you'd rather curl up on the couch. It's earned with every conscious effort to prioritize your sleep, manage your stress, and say "no" to the habits that keep you stuck.

Are you ready to own your Type Zero lifestyle? To unlock the full power of your metabolic health and rewrite the script on your future? It's time to stop relinquishing your power and start taking control.

Your future starts *now*.

References

Source 1: https://www.myfooddata.com/articles/high-sugar-vegetables.php

Source 2: https://www.hsph.harvard.edu/news/press-releases/eating-whole-fruits-linked-to-lower-risk-of-type-2-diabetes/

Source 3: https://news.weill.cornell.edu/news/2015/06/food-order-has-significant-impact-on-glucose-and-insulin-levels-louis-aronne

Source 4: https://nutritionsource.hsph.harvard.edu/healthy-drinks/sugary-drinks/

Source 5: https://pmc.ncbi.nlm.nih.gov/articles/PMC6488513/

Source 6: https://urnow.richmond.edu/features/article/-/20787/whats-the-difference-between-sugar-other-natural-sweeteners-and-artificial-sweeteners-a-food-chemist-explains-sweet-science.html

Source 7: https://pmc.ncbi.nlm.nih.gov/articles/PMC10465821/

Source 8: https://www.sydney.edu.au/news-opinion/news/2016/07/13/why-artificial-sweeteners-can-increase-appetite.html

Source 9: https://pubmed.ncbi.nlm.nih.gov/24243632/

Source 10: https://journals.lww.com/cardiovascularendocrinology/fulltext/2021/09000/the_acute_vs__chronic_effect_of_exercise_on.1.aspx

Source 11: https://www.diabetes.co.uk/body/visceral-fat.html

Source 12: https://pmc.ncbi.nlm.nih.gov/articles/PMC11013274/

Source 13: https://pmc.ncbi.nlm.nih.gov/articles/PMC7849939/

Source 14: https://pmc.ncbi.nlm.nih.gov/articles/PMC2084401/

Source 15: https://pmc.ncbi.nlm.nih.gov/articles/PMC5070477/

Source 16: Foster, R. G., & Kreitzman, L. (2014). The rhythm of rest and excess: Timing of food intake, sleep, and metabolism. *Cell Metabolism, 19*(5), 759–767. https://doi.org/10.1016/j.cmet.2014.04.011

Source 17: Burgess, H. J., Fogg, L. F., & Wing, J. K. (2015). Inconsistent sleep patterns disrupt insulin sensitivity and increase risk for type 2 diabetes. *Journal of Clinical Endocrinology & Metabolism, 100*(6), 2225–2232. https://doi.org/10.1210/jc.2015-1213

Source 18: Kohsaka, A., Laposky, A. D., Ramsey, K. M., Estrada, C., & Bass, J. (2006). High-fat diet disrupts behavioral and molecular circadian rhythms in mice. *Cell Metabolism, 4*(5), 309–319. https://doi.org/10.1016/j.cmet.2006.09.003

Source 19: Spiegel, K., Leproult, R., & Van Cauter, E. (2009). Impact of sleep debt on metabolic and endocrine function. *The Lancet, 354*(9188), 1435–1439. https://doi.org/10.1016/S0140-6736(99)01376-8

Source 20: Tasali, E., Leproult, R., & Van Cauter, E. (2008). Sleep restriction in healthy young men: Impact on glucose regulation and insulin sensitivity. *Journal of Clinical Endocrinology & Metabolism, 93*(6), 2454–2459. https://doi.org/10.1210/jc.2007-2637

Source 21: Gangwisch, J. E., Malaspina, D., & Boden-Albala, B. (2007). Sleep duration as a risk factor for diabetes mellitus in a large U.S. sample. *Sleep, 30*(9), 1147–1153. https://doi.org/10.1093/sleep/30.9.1147

Source 22: Mullington, J. M., Haack, M., Toth, M., & Meier-Ewert, H. K. (2009). Sleep loss and inflammation. *Sleep and Biological Rhythms, 7*(1), 38–43. https://doi.org/10.1111/j.1479-8425.2009.00324.x

Source 23: Kivimäki, M., Virtanen, M., Vahtera, J., Elovainio, M., & Kouvonen, A. (2006). Work stress in the etiology of coronary heart disease—A meta-analysis. *Scandinavian Journal of Work, Environment & Health, 32*(6), 441–446. https://doi.org/10.5271/sjweh.1054

Source 24: Chaput, J. P., Drapeau, V., Gaudreau, H., & Després, J. P. (2013). Sleep duration and quality and their association with obesity, diabetes, and cardiovascular risk factors. *Current Diabetes Reviews, 9*(3), 171–183. https://doi.org/10.2174/1573399811309020011

Source 25: Khan, A., Khattak, K. N., & Anderson, R. A. (2013). Cinnamon improves insulin sensitivity in a dose-dependent manner in healthy adults. *Journal of Medicinal Food, 16*(1), 77–83. https://doi.org/10.1089/jmf.2012.0258

Source 26: Hirshkowitz, M., Whiton, K., Albert, S. M., et al. (2015). National Sleep Foundation's sleep time duration recommendations: methodology and results of the 2015 study. *Sleep Health, 1*(1), 40–43. https://doi.org/10.1016/j.sleh.2014.12.010

Source 27: Panahi, Y., Darvish, M., & Sahebkar, A. (2013). Curcumin as an adjunct to antidiabetic drugs: A review. *Diabetes Care, 36*(6), 1117–1124. https://doi.org/10.2337/dc13-0156

Source 28: How to Make a Turmeric Latte (Golden Milk)

Ingredients:

- 1 cup unsweetened almond milk (or any milk of your choice)
- 1 teaspoon turmeric powder (or 1-inch piece of fresh turmeric, grated)
- ½ teaspoon cinnamon (optional, for flavor)
- Pinch of black pepper (to enhance curcumin absorption)
- ½ teaspoon honey or stevia (optional, for sweetness)
- ½ teaspoon coconut oil or ghee (optional, for added richness and absorption)

Instructions:

1. In a small saucepan, combine the almond milk, turmeric, cinnamon, and black pepper. Stir well.
2. Heat over medium-low heat, whisking constantly, until it's warmed through (but not boiling).
3. Once it's heated, add sweetener (optional) and coconut oil (optional). Stir until everything is blended well.
4. Pour into a mug, give it a final stir, and enjoy your warm, golden goodness!

Source 29: Yin, J., Li, Y., & Han, T. (2008). The hypoglycemic effects of berberine in type 2 diabetes mellitus: A systematic review. *Metabolism, 57*(5), 535–539. https://doi.org/10.1016/j.metabol.2007.12.004

Source 30: Barbagallo, M., & Dominguez, L. J. (2010). Magnesium and aging. *The Journal of Clinical Endocrinology & Metabolism, 95*(5), 2031–2037. https://doi.org/10.1210/jc.2009-1885

Source 31: How to hit the 250–500 mg daily target for magnesium through food:

Leafy Greens:

- Spinach (cooked): 1 cup of cooked spinach provides around 157 mg of magnesium.
- Swiss chard (cooked): 1 cup of cooked Swiss chard provides about 150 mg of magnesium.
- Collard Greens (cooked):
  Sure, you *could* eat 5 cups of collards for 250 mg of magnesium—but a better idea is to combine 2 cups of collards (~90 mg), ½ cup quinoa (~60 mg), and 1 oz pumpkin seeds (~150 mg), and voila: magnesium goal crushed.

Nuts and Seeds:

- Almonds: 1 ounce (about 23 almonds) provides around 80 mg of magnesium.
- Pumpkin seeds: 1 ounce (about ¼ cup) provides around 150 mg of magnesium.
- Cashews: 1 ounce (about 18 cashews) provides about 74 mg of magnesium.

Whole Grains:

- Quinoa (cooked): 1 cup provides about 118 mg of magnesium.
- Brown rice (cooked): 1 cup provides around 84 mg of magnesium.
- Oats (cooked): 1 cup provides about 61 mg of magnesium.

Source 32: Packer, L., et al. (2011). "Alpha-lipoic acid and its role in improving insulin sensitivity and reducing blood sugar levels." *Journal of Clinical Investigation, 121*(5), 1725–1733.

Source 33: Food Sources of Alpha-Lipoic Acid (ALA):

1. Spinach (1 cup cooked) – Contains about 0.1 to 0.2 mg of ALA.
2. Broccoli (1 cup cooked) – Contains about 0.1 to 0.2 mg of ALA.
3. Brussels sprouts (1 cup cooked) – Contains about 0.1 mg of ALA.
4. Tomatoes – A small amount, but still a source of ALA (less than 0.05 mg of ALA per cup).
5. Organ meats (such as liver, kidney) – These are the richest sources of ALA (1 to 2.5 mg of ALA per 100 grams / 3.5 oz).
6. Yeast – Particularly found in brewer's yeast (0.5 mg of ALA per tablespoon).

Source 34: Anderson, R. A., & Polansky, M. M. (2007). Chromium supplementation improves insulin sensitivity in people with type 2 diabetes. *Diabetes Technology & Therapeutics, 9*(6), 579–586. doi:10.1089/dia.2007.0063

Source 35: Zhang, X., Li, S., Ma, J., & Sun, X. (2016). Chromium supplementation reduces blood sugar levels in individuals with insulin resistance: A randomized, double-blind, placebo-controlled trial. *Journal of Clinical Endocrinology & Metabolism, 101*(8), 3211–3217. doi:10.1210/jc.2016-2124

Source 36: Foods rich in chromium include:

1. Broccoli – 1 cup of cooked broccoli contains approximately 22 mcg of chromium.
2. Grapes – A serving of 1 cup of grapes provides about 8–10 mcg of chromium.
3. Whole wheat – 1 slice of whole wheat bread contains about 10 mcg of chromium.
4. Green beans – 1 cup of cooked green beans contains around 2–3 mcg of chromium.
5. Potatoes – 1 medium-sized potato (with skin) contains around 2–3 mcg of chromium.
6. Meat – A 3-ounce serving of lean beef or chicken provides around 2–3 mcg of chromium.
7. Eggs – 1 large egg has about 0.3–1 mcg of chromium.
8. Garlic – 1 clove of garlic provides about 0.4 mcg of chromium.
9. Mushrooms – 1 cup of cooked mushrooms contains around 2 mcg of chromium.

Source 37: https://pubmed.ncbi.nlm.nih.gov/14694010/?

Source 38: Arjmandfard D, Behzadi M, Sohrabi Z, Mohammadi Sartang M. *Effects of apple cider vinegar on glycemic control and insulin sensitivity in patients with type 2 diabetes: A GRADE-assessed systematic review and dose–response meta-analysis of controlled clinical trials.* **Frontiers in Nutrition.** 2025;12:1528383. doi:10.3389/fnut.2025.1528383

Source 39: https://nutrition.bmj.com/content/early/2024/01/18/bmjnph-2023-000823?

Source 40:

https://academic.oup.com/jcem/article/99/1/178/2836224?

Source 41: https://www.verywellhealth.com/health-benefits-of-zinc-8710684?

Source 42: Zinc-Rich Foods and Their Amounts:

Here are some foods that are high in zinc, along with the approximate zinc content per serving:

1. Oysters (3 ounces): 74 mg of zinc
2. Beef (3 ounces): 7 mg of zinc
3. Chicken (3 ounces): 2.7 mg of zinc
4. Pumpkin Seeds (1 ounce): 2.2 mg of zinc
5. Cashews (1 ounce): 1.6 mg of zinc
6. Chickpeas (1 cup, cooked): 2.5 mg of zinc
7. Lentils (1 cup, cooked): 1.3 mg of zinc
8. Quinoa (1 cup, cooked): 2 mg of zinc
9. Oats (1 cup, cooked): 1.1 mg of zinc

How Much Do You Need to Eat?

To reach the 20 to 40 mg per day recommended dose, you'd need to consume quite a bit of zinc-rich food. For instance:

- Oysters: Eating just one 3-ounce serving of oysters will give you more than the daily recommended dose, providing 74 mg of zinc.
- Beef: If you ate about 6 ounces of beef (roughly two 3-ounce servings), you would get around 14 mg of zinc, which is half the recommended dose.
- Pumpkin seeds: You'd need to consume about 10 ounces (roughly 2/3 cup) of pumpkin seeds to get 22 mg of zinc.

Source 43: https://care.diabetesjournals.org/content/26/5/1619.full.pdf?

Source 44: Food Sources of Omega-3s:

- Fatty Fish (e.g., salmon, mackerel, sardines, herring)
    - 3 ounces of cooked salmon = approximately 1,000 milligrams of omega-3s
    - Mackerel and sardines are also excellent sources, with a similar amount of omega-3s per 3 ounces.
- Chia Seeds
    - 1 ounce (about 2 tablespoons) = approximately 5,000 milligrams of omega-3s.
- Flaxseeds (ground is best for absorption)
    - 1 tablespoon = 2,350 milligrams of omega-3s.
- Walnuts
    - ¼ cup = 2,300 milligrams of omega-3s.
- Hemp Seeds
    - 3 tablespoons = about 6,000 milligrams of omega-3s.
- Algal Oil (a plant-based source of omega-3s)
    - 1 teaspoon (depending on the brand) can provide around 500–1,000 milligrams of DHA, a form of omega-3 that's great for health.

How Much Do You Need to Eat to Reach the Effective Dose?

To reach the recommended 1,000–2,000 milligrams per day, you could eat the following:

- Salmon: One 3-ounce serving (roughly the size of a deck of cards) provides about 1,000 mg of omega-3s. You'd need about 1–2 servings per day to hit your goal.

- Chia Seeds: A 2-tablespoon serving gives you 5,000 mg—so, you'd be set with just one serving per day!
- Flaxseeds: You'd need about 1 tablespoon of ground flaxseeds per day to reach around 2,350 mg.
- Walnuts: A ¼ cup serving is about 2,300 mg, so a small handful daily could meet your goal.

About the Author

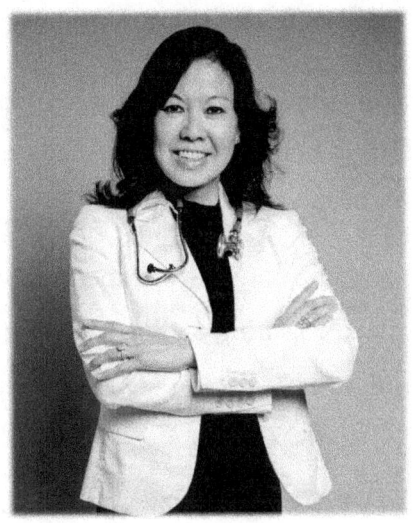

Dr. Mary Ann Martin is a board-certified Endocrinologist, Executive Health Coach, Speaker and Author. Known as Dr. Hormone Hacker, she disrupts our traditional, broken health care system and guides people on prevention & well care, not sick care. She is passionate about bridging the healthcare gap by helping people understand and balance their hormones, achieve a healthy body composition, prevent and reverse chronic diseases, and optimize their health proactively and holistically.

Facebook: https://www.facebook.com/maryann.martin.374549
Website: drhormonehacker.com

Ready to Rewrite Your Story?

Reading my journey was just the beginning - now it's YOUR turn.

If you're tired of the guessing game, frustrated by the one-size-fits-all advice, or scared of slipping into full-blown diabetes... I'm here to help you take control ...right now.

- ☑ Get a comprehensive hormone + metabolic lab panel
- ☑ Receive personalized coaching on nutrition, fitness, and lifestyle
- ☑ Crack the code of your body and step into your strongest, most energized self

As a double board-certified Endocrinologist (voted Best in Nevada), I've seen firsthand how powerful lifestyle medicine can be. It changed my life, and it can change yours too!

Spots are limited because I go deep with every client.
Don't wait for the diagnosis. Prevent it. Reverse it. Live fully.

Head to drhormonehacker.com
to book your breakthrough session now.
Let's hack your hormones and reclaim your health—together.

Dr. Mary Ann Martin
aka Dr. Hormone Hacker

www.ingramcontent.com/pod-product-compliance
Lightning Source LLC
Chambersburg PA
CBHW061704120626
46550CB00003B/1081